FREEDOM FROM FOOD

A Quantum Weight Loss Approach

PATRICIA BISCH, MA, MFT

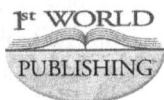

1st WORLD
PUBLISHING

Published by 1stWorld Publishing
1100 North 4th St., Fairfield, Iowa 52556
tel: 641-209-5000 • fax: 641-209-3001
web: www.1stworldpublishing.com

First Edition

LCCN: 2007931205
SoftCover ISBN: 978-1-4218-9986-2
HardCover ISBN: 978-1-4218-9987-9
eBook ISBN: 978-1-4218-9988-6

MEDICAL DISCLAIMER

The information drawn from the Freedom From Food process and the conclusions drawn thereon are the result of Patricia Bisch's personal and professional observations and interpretations through working with people and the process for over 30 years, along with her own personal healing. The information and suggestions for its use contained in this book are not intended to be a substitute for appropriate medical treatment. The information provided herein does not constitute medical advice. The information contained herein is provided for educational and instructional purposes only and is not offered as a prescription for the treatment of physical and mental illness. The use of any techniques described herein without the proper consultation with a health care professional is expressly discouraged. In the event that a reader undertakes to utilize the techniques without proper consultation with the appropriate health care professional, the author and publisher hereby expressly disclaim any responsibility for any harm incurred as a result.

Always consult your health care professional when confronted with a serious health problem. Any conditions, predispositions or allergies relative to food should be disclosed to the appropriate health care professional and considered prior to implementing any of the techniques described herein. Failure to consult a health care professional or to heed the advice of any health care professional is a liability that rests solely with the reader.

Adherence to the guidelines described herein does not insure successful outcomes in every case. The methods described herein are not inclusive of all accepted methods of care reasonably directed to the same result. The ultimate judgment regarding the appropriateness of any specific procedure, therapy or referral rests with the individual after proper consultation with the appropriate health care professional and viewed in light of all circumstances presented by an individual case.

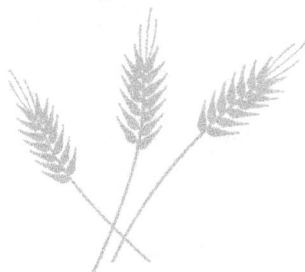

TESTIMONIALS

"Freedom From Food is about learning to nurture myself and my body from a true place. It's about once and for all clearing the 'food issue' and having the freedom and the power to live the life of my dreams now. It's about enjoying whatever food I might want to eat as never before. There really are no words to express the extent of this miraculous, transformational work. I feel very blessed to have found Patricia. Freedom From Food is now at the core of my spiritual practice."

"Absolutely the most extraordinary group 'nourishment' I've ever experienced! Puts everything in your life in perspective."

"What this program taught me was a new mindset. It is so amazing not to beat myself up anymore. I used to be the first one to make fun of myself or point out what I perceived to be my bodily flaws. I spent so much time putting myself down. The most valuable thing that I learned from Freedom From Food was not to give food power. It just doesn't even enter my mind. I eat what I want and as much as I want. What drives me now is what makes me feel healthier. I don't always make the healthiest choices in the food I eat, but the choice not to give the food power or beat myself up is the healthiest thing I have ever done. This program has changed my life.

FFF has given me Freedom, period. It's amazing that when I became free from the obsession of food, I had much more time to be productive in other areas of my life. We are usually not aware of all the negative talk we have created in our heads until we are given the gift of Patricia Bisch and this program. This is the miracle we have all been searching for."

～

"It is 20 years later that I am sharing my thoughts about the Freedom From Food program. I am still feeling healed with no desire to go on a diet or weigh myself. For me it was really a mental healing as well as a physical healing. I was always obsessive-compulsive about my body and consumed with the problem of weight and overeating. I was a fanatical workout person. I was in the gym 6 days a week doing weights and aerobics plus running, biking and stairs. I could be classified as an exercise bulimic. I would even exercise at night at weird hours. I felt fat and full. I always had to be on top of it. I was so upset and consumed with my body, always asking friends if I looked fat. I was afraid that I had to really keep controlled or I would blow up and never stop. A very big part of my life was spent dealing with this issue. I felt enslaved by food and weight. I was afraid that if I got fat, I would not be loved, and I knew I would hate myself. I felt I was not good enough. I was obsessed with my legs and thighs. I was always off balance eating and dieting, always looking and checking to see if I had gained weight. My eating consisted of binging and dieting over and over again. I was always on a diet.

When I took Patricia's class, the cycle broke, and I became free. I got an in-depth understanding that food has no power over me, and it has no power in and of itself. I remember looking at kids who eat and eat and never gain weight. We dissected in a logical way old beliefs about food. I still remember the concept we learned that full does not equal fat. I don't consciously think of the principles I learned anymore, but I know they are there in my consciousness.

I haven't weighed myself in over 20 years. I so well remember how weighing can trap a person. I remember being astounded that I didn't gain 20 pounds after eating hamburgers, french fries and sundaes. After that time, I exercised but not neurotically or compulsively, and I ate what I wanted. I would eat a lot at Thanksgiving or Christmas or parties and never gain weight. I found that my body would just balance out. I believe that the extra food will just dissolve in the ethers. You don't have to burn it off; it just goes away. I found I can even just lie in bed and it dissolves. It's like air; it just goes in and out. I now understand that matter has no substance. Consciousness is the source of my freedom."

—

"Freedom From Food is a powerful program that is shifting the paradigm around food and weight. It has made a tremendous contribution to the quality of my life by shifting my belief system about food permanently, and also by helping me see clearly that everything occurs in my outer world as a reflection of my beliefs. When I change my beliefs, I change my experience of that thing. I am fully responsible. Thank you Patricia Bisch for your brilliant and transformational work."

—

"It was 17 years ago that I was blessed to meet Patricia Bisch. My meeting with her most definitely comes under the heading of a miracle. Her education, or should I say reeducation, about food quite possibly saved my life. At the time of writing this, I am 47 years old. In my mid-20s, I developed an eating disorder. There were days when I just about starved myself and exercised like crazy, somewhere between 18–22 hours a week. At some point, my tongue was black, and I was told this was due to malnutrition. My hair started falling out, and I developed gum disease, also of course due to being malnourished. During those years, my life was a nightmare, and I was obsessed with dieting, calories, exercise, and feeling guilty when I thought I ate more than I should.

For the past 17 years, I have not once thought about how many calories are in something, have not once dieted and have not once obsessed about food. I am sorry to say I do not exercise very much, and for all of this time I have been my perfect weight. I am an American size 4. Being small boned, I just know from my dress size, what I see in the mirror and how I feel that I am my perfect weight. As one of my roommates says frequently, 'Boy you can eat,' and it is fantastic to be able to do so without any fear of gaining weight.

I suffered so very much with my eating disorder. I want to

encourage all of you to trust Patricia's knowledge and to trust in the process so that, if you are currently suffering, you can know that there is indeed 'light at the end of the tunnel.' You too can enjoy eating 'whatever you want, in whatever quantity you want and be your perfect weight.' I wish you all the very best of luck and many guilt-free meals in the future!"

———

"It has been 4 years since I have been healed from my weight problem and giving food my power. I recently went through some devastating events in my life, which makes this story even more incredible. My father got cancer, I am completely remodeling my house and I am facing some deep feelings of aloneness. I know that without having gone through this FFF program I would have gone up at least two clothes sizes. However, I find I am still losing weight and now am a size 2. I am living proof that the body/mind connection is so powerful."

———

"Thanks to Patricia and her extraordinary course, I have experienced over 5 years of living in my perfect proportion while being free from any concerns over how or what I should eat. I've forever banished the word *diet* from my vocabulary and I've made it a point to no longer listen to outside sources to know what is true for me. I came to Freedom From Food from a desperate place, where the power I gave food ruled much of my thinking. I spent over 20 years being obsessed with being thin and finding the so-called perfect diet plan that would get and keep me there. But, no matter what I tried, the results were temporary and my mind, body and valuable time consistently paid a price. Today, I can honestly say I am free from food!! Through Patricia's classes, I have discovered that our bodies were miraculously created to handle anything and will always fight for our perfect proportions—if we resist all negative thought patterns and manmade beliefs about food. This miracle has forever changed my life! I am free to eat whatever I want, whenever I want! I am free to experience the fullness of life in a way I used to only dream was possible!"

"Patricia and I spend about 3 or 4 nights a week together socializing. These evenings always include meals. While I have gone through and follow well-known weight loss programs, Patricia eats at least twice what I eat and whatever she wants. She basically eats all the time. She eats snacks that I rarely touch. She eats ice cream, which I have given up! Her weight miraculously stays the same, while I go up and down...mostly up! I use menopause as an excuse, but we're both the same age!"

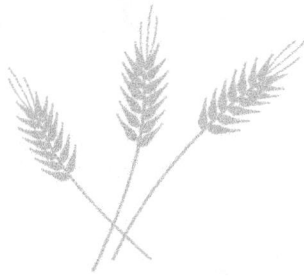

DEDICATION

I dedicate this book to my dear teacher of Eschatology, Nick Lentine, for his unending exuberance and immoveable stand for the goodness of life. Thank you for helping me heal my broken wing until I could fly.

To my mother, for seeing me and giving me spiritual roots.

To my son Keegan, for his incredible loving, warm, deep heart and for adding so much joy and music to my life.

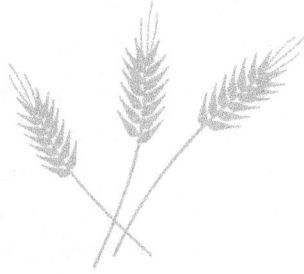

ACKNOWLEDGEMENTS

There are so many people that I wish to thank who have been instrumental in my process of birthing this book. It has been a 4-year labor of love to finish the actual writing. To begin with, I wish to thank Nick Lentine for his mastery as a teacher of Eschatology, for his wisdom, generosity, friendship and love. Thanks also to his wife, Nina Lentine, and family for graciously opening up their home to me for 8 years.

When it comes to endless hours of patience, endurance, dedication to the vision, professionalism and understanding, I wish to thank my main editor, Ann West. This book would not have come into form without her support. I would also like to thank editor Donna Beech who got me started on this book who lovingly held my hand in the beginning stages. Thanks to editor Cynthia Anderson for her additions and helpful encouragement to stand behind my work. Also, I thank editor Nancy Marriott for her wonderful polishing in the final stages of the manuscript as well as her encouragement and enthusiasm for this project.

I want to thank all those who have participated in the Freedom From Food classes and believe in this program. You have been a great source of inspiration for me. It is through watching your empowering transformations that I have been motivated to write this book. Special thanks to Jan Clinton for your unyielding dedication and support. Dennie LaTourelle, thank you for coaching and bringing your wisdom and understanding of myth to this course.

My gratitude extends to all of those special heart friends who put their magical editing touches on various chapters in the book and have loved me through this process: Robert Strock, Marilyn Levine,

Mary Kay Fry, Sharon Leeds, Melanie Hutton, Noell Grace, Mary Norris, Ruth Rapaport, Hannah Hunter, Lei Lacy, Julie Casal, Karin Chelsey, Sanda and Frank Jasper, Linda and Amy Levine, Barb Grant, the Berkowitz family and Anny Eastwood. Special thanks to the Bisch Family, Jeff, Keegan, Jason, Erica, Emma, Zachary, Keegan Bisch and Leah Metzger, Natalie and Coco Robinson, Wyatt Winborne, Lucas Rasovich, Billie and James MacLeod, Pearl Rafferty and the Lichtenstein family: grandmother Ester, mother Billie and father Irv and Lisa. I would also like to thank Rita and Gary Considine, Vito Sanzone, Cathy Highland, Magi Mygen, Patricia Diorio, Terri Apanasewicz, Joyful, Indu, Katya, Seppie Hope, Deborah, Tarra Walter, Nino and Sue for believing in this program. Also thanks to Karen Weingard, grandfather Abraham Berkowitz and Michael Beckwith for their spiritual inspiration. From Muscletone Village Studio, appreciation to Ira Ingber for his wonderful recording and mixing contributions on the *Freedom From Food* CD.

Thanks to Meganne Forbes for her exquisite watercolor picture, *The Body of Flowers,* in the third chapter. Thank you Benjamin Cziller for your wonderful work on the cover and to Jodi de Marcos for the photograph on the back cover. My deep appreciation goes to Candace B. Pert, Barbara Marx Hubbard, Judith Orloff, Barbara De Angelis and others who have endorsed this book and given it wings to fly. For all of those who may not be named specifically but have helped in any way, I thank you all from the bottom of my heart for helping me deliver this new consciousness into the world.

CONTENTS

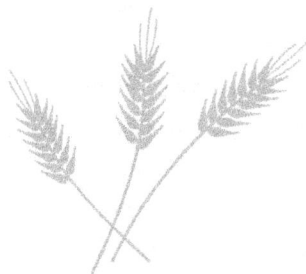

INTRODUCTION

The truth is that our bodies are rivers of intelligence, information and energy constantly renewing themselves in every second of their existence. Just as you cannot step into exactly the same river twice, you cannot inhabit the same flesh and bones for even a fraction of a second because, in every instant, you're literally creating a new body. You change your body more effortlessly, more spontaneously, and more expeditiously than you can change your clothes. In fact, right now, this very second, the body that you're using to read this book is not the same one you started out with a few minutes ago.

—Deepak Chopra, MD, *Perfect Weight*

The Freedom From Food (FFF) program delivers a revolutionary perspective and an unprecedented process for returning your body to its perfect proportion *without dieting*. This radical technology works with your consciousness to change the way food affects your body. The outcome is that you will be able to eat whatever you want, eat as much as you want and never gain weight.

Can You Change Your Body With Your Mind?

From my own personal healing and from experience in working with individuals and groups for 30 years, my answer to this question is *"YES"*! The advances made in quantum physics reveal that the material world is an optical illusion. We are not solely what we see. When my healing happened, this idea was not being discussed. Now quantum physicists have substantiated the body/mind connection. There is abundant scientific evidence that our thoughts and emotions directly affect our physical form.

The FFF process is aligned with Einstein's theory—everything in our world is energy slowed down to assume the appearance of matter. This matter is not fixed. Dr. Deepak Chopra, in his book *Perfect Weight*, confirmed that 99.999996 percent of our body is, in fact, empty space that changes with every breath we take. Although the world appears to be stationary to the naked eye and our bodies appear to be solid, we are constantly moving and fluctuating. By following the specific progression in the FFF program, you will experience how you are creating with your energy all the time and how you are affecting your body.

Through ancient knowledge, yogis have shown us extraordinary possibilities of what can be accomplished when you focus the mind to change the body. There are stories of yogis from the Himalayas who can submerge their bodies in subfreezing temperatures. The heat from their bodies melts snow up to 10 feet around while they stay at the normal temperature of 98.6 degrees Fahrenheit. To produce such feats, they train their minds with such methods as visualization, hypnosis and other methods that alter their energies and vibrations.

These same principles are available for you and me in our everyday life. Freedom From Food takes the body/mind concept out of mental theory or speculation and empowers you to demonstrate these universal laws on yourself. You will master how to change your physical form by changing your consciousness.

Freedom From Food has brought me, and many others, out of the devastating pain of food addiction and into an empowered place that is totally free from the bondage of food. The program shows how to remove permanently the veils of your mind that keep you from knowing your full strength and living in harmony in your body temple. If you dedicate yourself to this process, you too can live in a world where you can eat whatever you want, eat as much as you want and not gain weight.

Why Freedom From Food Is Different

Although other weight loss programs talk about the body/mind connection, they inevitably say or imply that the weight will come off only in conjunction with specific diet-related actions. FFF is different. It has no diet. It does not tell you to cut down your food intake or eat certain foods at certain times in a certain way. It does not deal with lowering calories, eating only when you're hungry, watching fats or carbohydrates, drinking large amounts of water, exercising or evaluating your body type. Although I feel that some of these elements are important for a balanced healthy life, it is possible to lose weight in a way that is completely separate from them.

FFF is unique in its purity, in the way it examines mind-over-matter principles and how they are integrally connected to weight (not health). To lose weight, it makes no difference whether you eat junk food or health food—either your mind can affect your body, or it can't. In this program, there are no catches.

I do not want to oversimplify what is needed to heal a food problem and to correct the misperception that what you eat affects your weight. This process is not for the faint of heart or the wishy-washy. To shift what your body does with food, you need an open mind, intense practice and the ability to hold a new consciousness for the rest of your life.

Intellectual knowledge is not enough. It is not about declaring, "Food makes me thin," on Monday and starting a new diet on Tuesday. The FFF process must be done on a weekly basis as directed by the guidelines at the end of each chapter. To anchor a new way of thinking permanently and eliminate unconscious, negative messages about food, you will need to make a commitment of at least 6–12 months.

Weight and Health

I want to be clear that I am not advocating in any way that it is advisable to eat junk food or unhealthy food, or to overeat and not exercise. I believe in being physically active and eating what is nourishing. Neither do I claim in any way to know what foods are healthy or unhealthy for you. I am making a definite distinction about the connection between food and weight, *not* food and health. For the latter, I recommend you follow professional, medical advice.

However, I have seen that deprivation makes forbidden foods only more desirable. Therefore, the path of this program is to neutralize the effects of *all food* on your weight. This gives you the freedom to choose what to eat, not because you might fear getting fat but for improving the quality of your life.

In Conclusion

The FFF program will teach you how to experience food as moving energy (*quantum physics approach*) instead of dense matter (*Newtonian physics approach*). The quantum approach makes available a different set of natural laws than the methods adopted by our diet-crazed world. The new paradigm is based on expanding your consciousness. *Consciousness* refers to your ability to be aware, to understand the subtleties of the physical and quantum worlds and to make this awareness a reality in daily life. The FFF methods bypass judgments that food is either "good" or "bad." Food—whether celery sticks or a jelly donut—is viewed as neutral energy that the mind directs according to your beliefs. Now you will have an opportunity to demonstrate these unique and exciting principles on yourself.

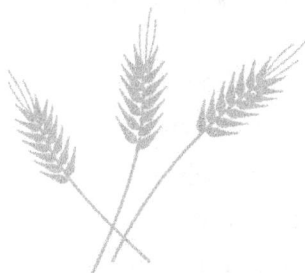

HOW TO USE THIS BOOK

Freedom From Food (FFF) is divided into five parts. The chapters within each part follow an essential progression to align your thinking and create a paradigm shift in the way food affects your body. For this reason, it is important that you read the chapters in order and do the practice sessions at the end of each chapter exactly as described. There are two CDs that are highly recommended to accompany the practice sessions and will greatly add to your success in this program. See the back of the book to order them.

Most examples in this book will use the pronoun *her* when referring to a person, although this program was also created for men. Therefore, as you read this book, please apply the appropriate gender.

I want to reinforce that this is not a quick-fix weight loss program. FFF is for people who have given up on all diet programs—those ready to try something new and willing to do whatever it takes to return to their perfect proportion. The miracle is that *once you have mastered the Keys to the process, you have the possibility of permanent freedom from the bondage of food and from being overweight.*

Outline of the Program

Part I: Why Freedom From Food? In Part I, you will be guided through two introductory chapters: Diets Don't Work and My Story. They are each followed by your first practice sessions.

Part II: The Four Mastery Keys. You will travel down a path guided by a Wise Woman, who will teach you the Four Mastery Keys that are essential to understand in order to heal yourself:

Key 1: The Body Heals Itself
Key 2: Mind Creates Matter
Key 3: Emotions Affect Your Body
Key 4: Food Is Energy

The Four Mastery Keys are reinforced by exercises that assist you to embody the concepts.

Part III: Empowerment Training: Preparation for 2-Week Healing. This training teaches you to become a *Warrioress*. It will take you far beyond just thinking thin. You will acquire skills to fight the dragons and mental saboteurs of doubt, fear and self-loathing that contribute to weight gain and keep you stuck in a negative cycle. You will learn how to hold a stand and how to focus long enough to actually create a change in the way your body processes food. You will see for yourself that if you are 100 percent vigilant and impeccable in how you think, you will be able to eat chocolate, bread and butter, or anything else, and it will not affect your weight. This requires you to step into a mastery level of consciousness in a way that you have never done before.

Part IV: Demonstration and Transformation. You will learn the incredible power and strength of your own mind! You will go through a trial by fire by doing a *2-Week Healing* on yourself. First you will create a Ceremony of Empowerment to make sure you are ready. Then you will be guided through steps where you will get on and off a scale and prove to yourself that you no longer gain weight from food. This process, which is the same one I went through 30 years ago, is designed to create a quantum shift in how food affects your body. As negative thoughts and deprivation diminish, so will your compulsion and obsession with food.

Part V: Follow-Up. In this part, you will learn how to *practice* and *support* your new consciousness. When you know beyond a shadow of a doubt that food does not make you gain weight, you have the possibility to start losing weight and return to your perfect proportion. Because consciousness creates, you are responsible for the thoughts you entertain from this point forward. As deprivation ceases, you naturally move into *Advanced Eating*. You will find yourself choosing foods that help you think more clearly, give you more energy and make you feel better. You won't gain weight if you don't eat this way, but as your healing progresses, you will be drawn to foods that enhance your quality of life.

Timeframe

The FFF program takes about *6–12 months* to complete. The preparation for the 2-Week Healing takes approximately 4 months, followed by 2–10 months of additional review, support and deepening of the practice. Doing the exercises in the practice session at the end of each chapter requires approximately 1 hour a week for individuals and 2½ hours a week for those meeting in a group, depending on the size of the group. This program is set up purposefully in the exact progression necessary to get the optimum results and to open the possibility for you to make a quantum leap to change your body.

The timeframe is based on the experiences of people who have worked the steps successfully. I have not found any short cuts, so I advise you not to jump ahead prematurely. Your mind may understand the material, but without the in-depth work provided by the exercises, you will gain nothing more than intellectual knowledge. During this program, I highly recommend that you receive professional help to clear out any emotional issues that may be affecting you. The FFF program is not a replacement for consistent psychological work.

Journaling

Keep a journal throughout the course. Jot down the things you relate to most strongly and make notes about questions that come up as you read this book. You can also use your journal to remember and track poignant things other people say, empowering thoughts you may have or messages from the past you know you need to address. Your journal is the record of your journey. It will be of great value when you do your 2-Week Healing and need to remember the program's essential principles.

Sacred Space

Create a sacred space in your home where you can write in your journal and reflect on your experiences in this program. You may decorate it with candles, sacred objects, pictures of yourself at your perfect weight, affirmations and the like. Whenever you pass by or spend time in your sacred space, it will remind you of your intentions and be a focal point for the new thoughts you are putting into your consciousness.

Inner Child Work

Do some Inner Child work every day. It is important for your Inner Child to feel that she can trust your Adult Self to protect and draw boundaries for her. Weight is often a protection against abuse, hurt or unwanted sexual advances. Your Inner Child may not release excess weight until she feels confident that your Adult Self will be there for her in the way that food has been—and her original parents have not. This relationship will grow over time. Here are two recommendations for how to work with her:

1. Listen to the Inner Child segment on the *Freedom From Food* CD with audible words.

2. Keep your journal by your side while you create a dialogue between your Inner Child and your Adult Self. Close your eyes and picture your Inner Child. Notice what expression is on her face. Tune into how her heart feels. Ask her the following questions:

How are you feeling today? (mad, sad, angry, glad, scared, anxious)
Where do you feel this in your body?

How do you feel about how I am taking care of you?

Is there something you need from me?

How are you feeling about the people in your life? (friends, family, relationships)

What kinds of things would be fun for you to do?

Here is an example of how to nurture your Inner Child (the relationship will build over time):

I am the Nurturing Parent within you. If you have any problem, you can talk to me. I'll be there for you any time you need me. I am here to listen to you—just to listen. Tell me what is going on with you. You are No. 1 to me. You are important. I believe in you. I believe you can do anything you want to do in this life. Whenever you need to, just call on me and I will be there for you. I love you.

Setting up an Individual Practice

If you are working individually, I recommend that you set aside about an hour each week to do the exercises at the end of each chapter. Prior to each session, give yourself additional time to read and digest the new material. It will take 1–4 weeks to complete each practice session, depending on the number of exercises required.

The sacred space you create in your house is a good place to do your weekly activities. Be sure you will be undisturbed for the time allotted. If you like, light a candle or incense to signify the beginning of your practice. At different times during your session, you might hold a stone, a feather, a crystal or another object of special significance on which to focus your thoughts. Begin by using the Opening Attunement, which you will find at the end of this chapter.

Then, simply follow the step-by-step instructions. Go along at your own pace and be sure not to rush through the exercises. Write the answers to all questions in your journal. You can do the dialogues that occur periodically by speaking both parts A and B aloud. This is just as effective as having another person do this with you.

Once again, I recommend that you take at least 4 months to complete the practice sessions, integrating the material fully before you begin the 2-Week Healing, the process described in Part IV of the program outline.

Setting up a Group

It can be helpful to work the FFF program in a group. Groups can be of any size, but the optimal number of members is no more than from six to eight. I recommend that FFF groups switch the leader every week. By alternating this role, everyone will get a chance to take part in the process.

In my experience, it is best if group meetings last no longer than 2–2½ hours. Before each session, read the chapter at least once and give it careful thought. Then when you meet, you will go through the exercises together and share your responses. It will take up to 4 weeks to complete each practice session, depending on the size of your group. I recommend that you take at least 4 months to complete the practice sessions before you begin the 2-Week Healing as described in Part IV. I have found that the following elements are essential to keep FFF groups running smoothly:

• **Talking Piece**—The talking piece can be anything—a stone, a feather, a crystal, a rattle. It is given to the person who has the floor. While someone is holding the talking piece, other group members need to place their attention and focus on that individual. The talking piece creates a space for deep listening to occur. It is a time not to think about what you're going to say but to give your full attention to the person speaking. There should be no cross talk and no comments after the person shares. Listen from your heart and look at the person.

Whatever your group chooses as a talking piece should be brought to every meeting. It is preferable that the talking piece be the same every week. The energy from each person holding this object will build up a vibrational resonance and imbue the piece with special meaning for the group.

- **Timekeeper**—Choose a timekeeper at each meeting. Timing is very important in any group where people share their deepest feelings and the most personal details of their lives. Without an agreement about how long each person will share, it is easy to have meetings where one person monopolizes the time. A timer eliminates the possibility of this awkward situation.

Most of the timing estimates throughout the book are for a group of six to eight. Feel free to adjust the time allotted each person to speak according to the size of your group.

- **Confidentiality**—Everything that is spoken about in the group needs to stay confidential among the members. The group must be a place of absolute safety, where people can share their deepest feelings and issues without fear. The way to create this kind of secure space is to treat each person's words with the compassion, respect and confidentiality you would want for yourself. If you do not agree, you need to speak about it before the group starts.

Attunements

Whether you are meeting individually or in a group, plan to begin and end each weekly session with an attunement. If you are working alone, attunements will connect you with your Higher Self as well as help you focus on the intention of each session.

In this program, we define an *attunement* as a specific group of words (sounds may be used also) that creates an invisible, synergistic field of union and resonance between group members or between an individual and the wisest part of herself. Because they carry a strong vibratory frequency, these words help create a receptive environment where new thoughts can grow. This field attends to the inner parts of an individual that need healing. Attunements can blend, harmonize and call forth various aspects of self (or forces outside of the self) to increase the possibility for a quantum leap in consciousness.

Note: In the sample attunement, I use the "Overlighting Angel" idea from my experience in Findhorn, an intentional community in Scotland that reflects a deep connection with nature and the Deva Kingdom. I call on the Overlighting Angel because I have always had my own connection with the angels and devas. However, please change this or any other parts of the attunements that might make you feel more comfortable.

Sample Opening Attunement for Individuals

I call in the Overlighting Angel of Food and Weight, who holds the knowledge of the universal principles and truths about food. I take a deep breath in and open the top of my head, open my mind and become receptive.

I call in my Higher Self, who knows, on the deepest level, that I am one with all of creation; that I hold within my being all of the ancient and scientific principles that exist everywhere and that I have already inside of me all the answers I am seeking.

Next, I call in the Warrioress part of myself, who is strong and fierce and alert, and who can draw impenetrable boundaries around all that I hold sacred.

Now, I call in, very tenderly, the part of myself that needs healing around my weight issue. Tuning in, I listen to what this part is feeling—mad, sad, happy, angry, fearful (pause). Now, I send love from my heart to this aspect of myself. I thank this part for having the courage to show up. I hold the intention that I will get exactly what I need for my weight healing today.

Sample Closing Attunement for Individuals

I thank the Overlighting Angel of Food and Weight for being with me today. I thank my Higher Self and my Warrioress for being here. I thank the part of myself that needed healing today for having the courage to show up and be present. I know that the seeds that I have planted today in my consciousness are already growing on a conscious, unconscious and subconscious level, and that my body has already begun its journey back to my perfect proportion as I set the intention for this to be so.

Sample Opening Attunement for Groups

We call in the Overlighting Angel of Food and Weight, who holds the knowledge of the universal principles and truths about food. We take a deep breath in and open the top of our heads, open our minds and become receptive.

We call in our Higher Selves, who know, on the deepest levels, that we are all essentially One; that we hold within our being all of the ancient and scientific principles that exist everywhere and that we have already inside of us all the answers we are seeking.

Next, we call in the Warrioress part of us, who is strong and fierce and alert, and who can draw impenetrable boundaries around all that we hold sacred.

Now, we place in the center of the circle, very tenderly, the part of each one of us that needs healing around this weight issue. We thank this part for having the courage to show up today and let itself be seen. We tune to what this part is feeling—mad, sad, happy, angry, fearful—and silently listen to what is going on with her (pause). Now, send love from your heart to this part of yourself. Then, breathe that love into the center of the circle (pause). Let us each hold the intention that every person in the group will get exactly what they are needing today.

Take a deep breath in as we open our minds, bodies and hearts, joining together in a common purpose—knowing that miracles can happen when members of a group hold the same intention. A beautiful synergy of the whole can happen that is more than the sum of its parts. So let us take a few moments in silence to create a resonant, receptive field by connecting, heart to heart, around the circle as we breathe, creating an opening and joining in one heart and one purpose for this group.

Sample Closing Attunement for Groups

We thank the Overlighting Angel of Food and Weight for being with us today. We thank our Higher Selves and our Warrioress for being a part of the circle. We thank the part of ourselves that needed healing today and had the courage to show up and be present. We know that the seeds that we have planted today in our consciousness are already growing on a conscious, unconscious and subconscious level, and that our bodies have already begun their journey back to our perfect proportions as we set the intention for this to be so.

In Conclusion

Review this chapter a few times before you start your weekly meetings. You cannot fill a vessel already full. Therefore, in the next chapter, Diets Don't Work, you will have a chance to clear your mind about any previous experiences that you have had from eating programs that have failed. Then you will be ready to fully take in the fresh new concepts of the FFF program.

PART I

WHY FREEDOM FROM FOOD?

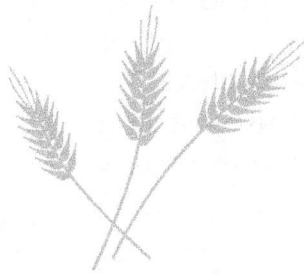

ONE

DIETS DON'T WORK

We are members of a fast-moving society, born and raised on instant gratification. We want fast cars, fast Internet connections, fast mail delivery, fast service and fast food. When we choose our diets, we pick the ones that promise weight loss—fast!

Diets have become a multimillion-dollar business. According to the International Food Information Council and Food Insight, dieters are spending an average of $30 billion a year on commercial weight loss programs.

For many of us, the need to take off extra pounds has literally become a matter of life and death. A front-page article of the *Los Angeles Times* on January 3, 2004, reported that obesity rates have risen 50 percent in the last decade. Excess weight and obesity contribute to the premature deaths of 300,000 Americans annually. According to the article, this is not far behind tobacco's yearly death toll of 430,000. Data from the 1999–2000 National Health and Nutrition Examination Survey (NHANES) indicate that about two thirds of adults in the United States are overweight (approximately 44 million) and 30.5 percent are obese.

Despite our best efforts to lose weight, and despite all the restrictive plans we try, statistics show that the weight reduction is temporary and the extra pounds usually return in a short time,

19

confirming that diets are ineffective. Clearly, a new solution is needed. I believe it is imperative that we start taking a different look at the devastating problem of overweight.

First, let's examine four basic reasons why diets don't work.

1. Diets Ignore Your Body's Natural Signals

Most of us learn early to ignore our body's natural signals. As babies, we know when we're hungry and when we're not. We reject food if we're not hungry and cry out for it when we are. But many parenting books, and the experts who write them, teach parents to override these natural instincts of infants and put them on an arbitrary feeding schedule.

After a few years, we are taught to eat only three meals a day and told we must finish everything on our plate whether we want it or not. We begin to get disconnected from our own inner authority and our capacity to listen to what we want to eat and when we want to eat it. We lose our whole ability to trust our own natural rhythms. Later we search for diets or regimens to tell us what and how much we should eat.

2. Diets Are Based on Losing

Diets are based on losing weight. What I have seen is that if I lose something, it is gone forever. If I find it again after a day, a week, a month or a year, it really wasn't lost; it was just temporarily misplaced.

In my experience, any weight I thought I had lost on a diet was always lurking nearby, ready to return the moment I took that first fatal bite. Weight gain was only a donut or a bag of chips away. What had taken so long to get rid of and demanded such grueling discipline came rushing back overnight, almost laughing at me for thinking I had ever lost it! This is why I feel that permanent weight loss must be accompanied by an entirely new consciousness and relationship with food, which a person continues for the rest of one's life. Most dieting is like putting duct tape over a hole in a boat. It is never going to work. It is not natural. Rather, we need to learn new ways that honor the body/mind connection.

3. Diets Don't Address the Underlying Issues

A diet alone does not address the psychological issues that are deeply connected to weight. People typically feel, consciously or unconsciously, that they are safer when they are heavier. Their weight has a psychological purpose. It serves as the boundary to protect them from harm and numb them from feeling pain they can't handle.

Often what happens on a diet is that people lose weight on the outside while still holding the consciousness and emotional insecurities of a fat person on the inside. The anxiety of being noticed and seen again out in the world makes them feel too vulnerable, and they put the extra pounds back on. There are many other psychological reasons why people gain weight, and we will address them in depth elsewhere in the book.

4. Diets Are Based on Deprivation

Most diets are based on deprivation, which makes you obsessed with what you can't have. If you are forbidden to eat chocolate, then chocolate seems to be the only thing you want. (In my case, candy bars and brownies topped my binge list.)

Our world has a plethora of delicious, succulent foods for us to eat and enjoy. These are literally the source of our nourishment and life. Restricting foods and limiting ourselves are unhealthy, unnatural behaviors, unless indicated otherwise by a medical professional. In the FFF program, you will learn a completely new paradigm about food. As you focus on how to change your consciousness, you will be able to eat whatever you want and not gain weight. There will be no deprivation and unhealthy binge eating will naturally subside.

You Are in Charge

Although you will not be on a diet in this program, you will need to give 100 percent of yourself to change your consciousness and confront old belief systems. During this time, you can expect to meet some shadowy, stuck parts of yourself. You are likely to find that your old ways of handling things are useless against some of the monsters that rear their ugly heads.

Sometimes you will find yourself caught between the old and the new, desperately wanting to point the finger of blame toward someone else for being in an uncomfortable place. At those times, you must *take responsibility to reverse the finger that is pointing out so it instead points back at you*.

In the end, you are responsible for your own healing process and the results you get from this program. You must understand that your healing journey is unique and that you may have to alter this process to fit some of your specific needs. Once again, do not go against anything that a medical doctor or other professional has advised for you.

Take It One Week at a Time

Some people will insist on changing their eating patterns immediately after starting this book. This is part of the quick-fix diet mentality I mentioned. *Trust me when I tell you that you are not ready to do that.* There is a good reason that this course takes 6–12 months. In my experience, you must have a deep understanding, focus and conviction before your cells will rearrange and you will be able to eat whatever you want and not gain weight.

Remember, it takes a rock climber a lot of time to learn the necessary skills before she actually climbs the mountain. Therefore, I recommend that you follow the progression of the course and do not alter your eating habits at this stage. I will let you know later on in the book when it is advantageous to try making some changes. For now, your job is to start opening and expanding your mind to receive the new ideas that are being presented. Let yourself put away any last remnants of diet mentality as you prepare to take this extraordinary FFF journey.

PRACTICE SESSION 1

Congratulations! You are ready to start the in-depth journey of *Freedom From Food.* I recommend that you review the sections called Setting up an Individual Practice and Setting up a Group in "How to Use This Book." For groups decide who will be this week's group leader and time keeper.

Visual Aid: Each chapter has a few key words that reinforce the active principle. On a piece of paper, write the guiding words and place them as a visual reminder in front of you. For groups, place this paper in the center of the circle. Each week you will add another sign with new key words. For this chapter, the sign will say:

~ Diets Don't Work ~

1. Opening Attunement (see sample on p. 13 or p. 14)

If you so desire, light a candle to mark the opening of the session. I recommend that you play the subliminal *Freedom From Food* CD quietly in the background during the attunement (see order information at the end of the book, p. 231).

2. Check-In (2–3 Minutes)

For Individuals: Write a page or more in your journal, checking in with yourself and answering the question that follows.

For Groups: Allow a 2–3-minute check-in per person. Answer the question that follows. (Be sure to pass the talking piece and use a timer.)

• What drew you to this program? (Also, speak a little about yourself.)

3. Break

4. Questions

For Individuals: Take as long as you wish to journal about each of the following questions. Then reread the answers you wrote.

- Do you feel that you deserve to be thin?

- What diets have you tried that didn't work?

- Have you given up on dieting?

- What fears do you have about going through this process?

For Groups: Go through the questions above one by one. Add the following question: What are your fears about being in the group? First, take 5 minutes to write in your journal your answers to the questions. Then go around the group to hear each person's response one question at a time. (Your timekeeper should allow each person 2 minutes to speak.) When everyone has had a chance to speak, go on to the next question.

5. Homework

This week, your homework assignment is to do the following:

a. Journal—Write down what you're feeling right before you eat, every time you eat, for one week. DO NOT change what you are eating. The only thing you will alter is to notice what you are feeling right before you put any food into your mouth. It may surprise you to notice the variety of things you feel when you eat—bored, stressed, anxious, rejected, sad, fearful, happy and so forth.

Here's an example. You are about to eat some chocolate chip cookies. Before you eat them, tune into the feelings going on inside and write them down. Maybe you feel anxious and realize that you are concerned about an important meeting you are about to have. Make a note: "anxious—important meeting." Then you can eat the cookies or not—whatever you want to do is fine. Once again, this is not an exercise to make you stop eating but to observe your feelings before you eat.

b. Journal—Write down the beliefs you are holding onto about food and weight. For example: I believe I need to exercise every day or I will gain weight. I believe people gain weight after age 40, especially women during menopause. I believe my mother is overweight, so I will be too. The first step in healing these beliefs is to become aware of them. Do not expect them to change right away. Changing beliefs is a process, and you will be given many tools for transformation that will assist you as you proceed through this book.

c. (Optional) Skip ahead to the next practice session in Chapter 2 (for groups, choose one person to do this). Read Exercise 7 and, if you wish, prepare a tape in advance of the next session.

Reminder for groups: Choose a new leader for next week.

6. Appreciation

For Individuals: Write a few sentences in your journal about what most moved and inspired you in this chapter.

For Groups: Go around the circle. Speak about what most moved and inspired you in the meeting today.

7. Closing Attunement (see sample on p. 13 or p. 14)

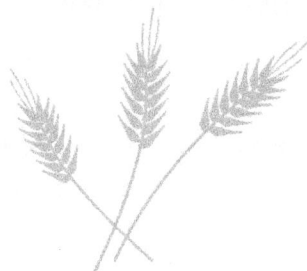

TWO

MY STORY

Food is the glue that holds my fragmented parts together so I look whole and no one can see I am really in pieces. Part of me knows that I am hiding in the shadows of my isolate world, where things are not as they seem on the outside. Inside, I'm loathing myself. I feel defective and just not good enough.

The outside world is beating me up emotionally. I don't feel that I have a buffer strong enough to shield me from the onslaught of predatory comments and critical judgments. There is so much fear inside of me. I feel shaky and nervous. My feelings have to go underground to make certain I don't get hurt anymore. I am too sensitive, too open and too raw. At the same time, I realize I have to be tough in this world if I want to survive. Food is my protector.

Like a loving parent, it shelters me from feeling unloved, anxious and out of control. No one can see the real me or detect my cover up. Like a phantom of the night, I fear if people really know how vulnerable and afraid I am, or witness the way I use food, they won't want to be my friend. I am eating to numb my pain and give myself the love I am so desperately needing. I feel so alone.

—Patricia Bisch (before healing)

How I Got Here

I was the apple of my dad's eye. To an idealizing child, my father was no less than perfect—a Martin Luther King-, Gandhi-type person. He taught me honor, integrity, truth and the highest of values. I was the star who could do no wrong, and he was the wind beneath my sails.

Although my father's love and attention empowered me, his affection also generated an unhealthy codependence. It impeded me from developing a real foundation of self-love. At age 5, when my younger sister was born, I felt eclipsed as he abruptly turned his entire attention and praise to her. She was standing in my light. This began to erode my perfect picture, creating fissures in my seemingly secure world. On the surface, I acted like it didn't matter, while inside I ached for his love to return. It never did.

I didn't have the capacity to figure out what had actually gone wrong. I spent countless hours in the secrecy of my own mind trying to understand. Children usually blame themselves, and so did I. When everyone exclaimed how beautiful my sister was, I deduced that my father had rejected me because I was ugly. This conclusion was the trigger for many years of haunting pain and self-hatred.

At the same time, to add to my emotional instability, my family moved from our warm and loving neighborhood to the cold austerity of Beverly Hills. I was the new kid on the block. From all appearances, my family was living the perfect life. My father was a prominent, successful doctor of the stars and the rich and famous. My dad's best friend was Burt Lancaster. People such as Dean Martin and Norman Lear were in his social circle. My mother was a beautiful socialite in designer dresses; she was filled with personality and charm. My sister was crowned the Homecoming Queen. And I played the role of the head cheerleader.

If you ask any of my friends from high school, they'll tell you that I was happy and popular in those years. My winning formula was to act like everything was great, and I played my role well. I was living a double life. On a deeper level, my pain and anger were beginning to surface—my body was gaining weight, my skin was breaking out and there was no one safe in whom to confide. I had all of the patterning of someone who was sexually abused, although it had never directly manifested.

At the same time, the American Dream our family appeared to be living cracked open and fell apart. My father seemed to have lost his love for my mother. He was becoming angry and domineering. My mother had changed from the charming, happy person I'd always known into someone who was depressed, in despair and unable to handle life.

Fighting, anger, betrayal and lies permeated our home and our hearts. When I found out my dad might be having an ongoing affair, the Gandhi-like picture I held of him disintegrated. It was hard seeing my mother and sisters in so much pain. Both parents were telling me conflicting stories. I could no longer tell truth from a lie. I was so confused. I remember the moment my father looked me in the eyes and lied. I was shattered in a way that I could no longer put the pieces back together and hold the illusion that I was happy. It was my fall from innocence. That is when I closed down my heart. Out of this barren reality my compulsion was born, and that's when food became the glue that replaced my father's love.

I started sedating my pain. To keep my act going, I began going on diets to repress my horrible anxiety and sadness. I was eating because the fear and anxiety were unmanageable. Sucked into the cycle of putting on weight and taking it off, I was in a never-ending battle of willpower, deprivation and collapse. Soon my whole self-esteem was wrapped up in how much I weighed. I went from diet to diet pills. My daily thoughts became consumed with the mad drive of losing weight. I was hoping to be beautiful enough once again to attract the love of a man who could make me feel like my father once had.

Enslaved by food, I was at the mercy of my compulsive overeating. It got to the point where every couple of days the dam of dieting would break, and I would have to binge. I would hit the liquor store like a bandit on the run. When I was fully into my binging, I would buy ice cream, candy bars, chips, little cakes and whatever else looked interesting. Then, once inside my car, I would eat it all until I felt full and in an altered state of oblivion.

As I devoured the food, my mind would fill with an endless barrage of self-hatred and hopeless thoughts. I would end up being so upset and ashamed that I would swear to myself I would start my diet the next day. Unfortunately, I could not stop repeating this cycle even though I had started going to a therapist. I had to eat to numb the pain; food was my morphine. My eating and dieting reeled out of control for many years to come.

Journey to Healing

I was crying out for help. There was no rest for my obsessive-compulsive mind. Healing my core sadness and hurt involved a team of loving souls to mend the deep wounds. I was delivered to the doors of three life-changing mentors. Each of these individuals became a gift bearer, holding the ground until I was able to shed my past and reclaim myself. They each held a piece of knowledge that guided me to the place where I was able to heal.

My journey first led me to Overeaters Anonymous (OA), where I met my sponsor. She was a gift bearer who taught me the spiritual practice (from OA) of turning my life over to a Higher Power. This gift was for the times when my thoughts would rapidly take a dive, spiraling down into a great abyss of negativity. My mind was like a room filled with snakes, and I did not know how to escape from my obsessive thinking. In those moments, life felt out of control, confusing and unmanageable.

My sponsor taught me to imagine that I was turning my problems over to a power that already had the wisdom and clarity to deal with uncomfortable situations. I would say, "OK, I am out of control. I cannot handle this problem or my life at this moment. I turn it over to You (my Higher Self, God, Truth, Nurturing Parent or whatever name feels comfortable) to take care of this issue in the highest way." I would visualize this happening. It gave my Inner Child something to hold onto when life got too much and she felt small and unable to handle things. I began to see that life did work out better when the little me let go of control and trusted. Although I never healed my food problem in OA, I found these lessons invaluable.

God bless my sponsor, wherever she is. I spoke to her for endless hours every day. She must have a permanent dent in her ear just from me. We talked about the most gut-wrenching, shame-filled subjects, secrets and feelings of inadequacy that I didn't want to admit to anyone. With the utmost patience and unwavering support, she gently helped me face my issues, grow up, and take charge of my life. I remember her saying that if I felt I had to punish myself for things I was feeling bad about, I could just as easily give myself a constructive punishment. She recommended that rather than stuffing myself and eating myself sick, I could clean out my closet. This idea and her numerous other suggestions helped slow down my obsessive, self-destructive thinking.

The next gift bearer I met was Robert Strock. If there are Guardian Angels in life, he certainly is one of mine. I was still very lost and depressed when I met him. I didn't know how to speak up to people or say that I felt differently. I was afraid I would be barraged by anger or have love withdrawn, as my father had done when I was a child.

With Robert, I finally had a friend who genuinely wanted to know my thoughts. It had been so difficult for me to realize that my father was being dishonest and didn't live by the ideals he had taught me. At the same time, it was deeply reassuring when Robert encouraged me to tell the truth and live with integrity despite what my father was doing. He helped me gain the courage to be authentic and go to a deeper level of emotional healing.

Robert would take my hand and look into my eyes. Because he was so present with me and I trusted him so much, I would often start to cry. All the pain that had accumulated in my heart for all those years would unravel. To this day, that still happens. Whether I am in my deepest darkest holes or celebrating my happiest moments, Robert is there, as I know he will be when I take my last breath. He is someone I can never thank enough. There is no doubt why he became an incredible therapist, beloved teacher to so many and my best friend.

Robert in turn led me to my third gift bearer, Nick Lentine, by inviting me to visit the spiritual class he taught, called Eschatology. Nick would later become the mentor who helped me find the way to change my relationship with food.

For the next 8 years, I studied with him how to heal all forms of disease by altering specific thoughts and emotions. Although I had improved, I was still dealing with my core issues of sadness, disillusionment and self-loathing. Nick was a reassuring force with boundless enthusiasm, always telling me life was good and that I had the ability to affect my circumstances. Ever so slowly, the class was beginning to thaw me out, as if I had been frozen. Nick's optimism started giving me the hope that I had lost so long ago. His joy slowly allowed me to rediscover my own childhood wonder and excitement for life.

The Healing Happens

I finally decided it was time that I prove to myself whether or not the theoretical knowledge I was learning could actually work. I wanted to face my wound or disease of compulsive overeating and really try to heal it. I approached Nick after class one day and told him my struggles with food. He asked, "Well, why don't you just stop eating?"

I'm sure all of you who are out-of-control eaters will have a good laugh. People who don't have this problem come up with statements like this in an innocent way—as if we haven't thought of that! Another thing they say is, "Have you looked in the mirror lately? You seem to have gained weight." As if we don't look in the mirror and feel the self-loathing about it every single day! What are people thinking?

I educated Nick and told him that a true compulsive eater was like an addict. I explained that I had no control over my eating. I was a junk food junkie. (There are overweight people who eat only healthy food or eat very little and still gain weight.)

Nick sat me down and told me what he wanted me to do. He asked me to write a meditation containing many of the principles about the body/mind connection that I had been studying. Also, he wanted me to get on a scale and note what I weighed at the beginning of this process. It was time to prove to myself the power of my thoughts. He said, "I want you to read this meditation 10 minutes a day, every day for 2 weeks. I want you to eat whatever you want, whenever you want it. At the end of 2 weeks, you will get back on the scale and see that you have not gained weight." (You too will go through a similar process in another chapter.)

This was a scary proposition. Although I was only about 30 pounds overweight, I was at my highest weight, at the peak of my binging activity and eating out of control compulsively. I knew this might mean a pint of ice cream a night and all my favorite liquor store junk food in endless quantities. I decided I was just going to do it anyway. I was so depressed and out of control, what did I have to lose? I trusted Nick completely.

I got on the scale the next morning, noted what I weighed and then put it away as instructed. For 2 weeks, I must admit I ate ravenously all the foods of which I had deprived myself. I also read my meditation for 10 minutes as I was told to do. I did not look back with doubt when I was doing this. I just ate and did what I was told.

In 2 weeks, I got back on the scale, and I had not gained any weight! This completely blew my mind!! Yes, of course, I understood theoretically what had happened. I understood the body/mind connection and the technology that had created this change. However, until then, I had only known these principles intellectually.

Looking down at the scale, I knew that it would have normally shown that I had gained 10–12 pounds after a 2-week binge. Now it was saying I had not gained any weight! I had transmuted this food with my thoughts. I knew something profound and life changing had just happened and that I would never be the same.

I had just experienced a miracle, an epiphany that proved to me

I could change my body system—with intention and extreme focus. I assume that I also had shifted my metabolism, since I was no longer gaining weight no matter what I ate. To me this was on the same level as healers who change cancer cells to normal cells or yogis who can put a knitting needle through their arm by focusing and holding a certain consciousness. But this was me, not a yogi, just a regular person.

I then decided that if my mind could keep me from gaining weight, why couldn't I direct my intention and focus to lose weight? That would seem to follow logically. Therefore, I changed my meditation to include the idea that I would lose weight. I continued to eat whatever I wanted, whenever I wanted it. To my utter surprise, it worked! And it kept on working over the course of about 6 weeks until I was at my perfect weight. I was awed! I will never forget the moment when I looked down at the scale and had lost weight after eating so much food.

I don't know if you have ever experienced something like this—something that goes beyond your understanding and creates a quantum shift in your body and mind. To me, even though I understood the principles that enabled this shift to occur, it still felt like a miracle! I have never lost the feeling of "Wow!" which comes when something of this magnitude occurs. I have never forgotten those moments when I looked down on the scale and understood, on a profound level, the power that my mind had on my body. I began to realize the far-reaching effects and unlimited possibilities for transformation this would have on my whole life. It has been 30 years since then, and I have never gained back the weight.

In Conclusion

Because I knew that my epiphany was a unique and important gift, I felt strongly that it had been given so I could help other people with the horrible, debilitating problem of compulsive overeating. It was with this in mind that I decided I must figure out the components of what had happened to me, and then I could teach others. From that point on, I began in earnest to create the Freedom From Food program.

It is my heartfelt wish to pass on this miracle and technology to those of you who are suffering as I did. I know we each have individual stories that carry our wounds. I know the devastating pain and hurt of being a compulsive overeater. If I can heal myself, I know that you can, too. You are not doomed to be affected by this problem all your life.

For some, this book may hold valuable keys on your path to healing and, if so, I am grateful to assist in that. For others, this information might be the last piece of the puzzle, as it was for me, on a long and difficult journey. I share my experience with you not as a scientist, or a medical professional, but as someone who has healed herself and helped many others over the years.

I recognize that this book is asking you to open up and expand into some new concepts that sometimes go beyond the confines of conventional thought. For example, I am respectful of today's study of genetics and differing views about whether people have a slow or fast metabolism based on their family of origin. However, I am not an expert on the subject, and this book is written from a different perspective that seems to work outside the confines of these ideas. Much to my own amazement, I have seen that the mind, when it fully embraces the FFF concepts, does have the possibility to influence and change the way the body processes food despite predisposed limitations.

I do not want to imply that this book is the only way to heal or that I have all the answers. There is a great mystery in life and our bodies that is still being unfolded. I have full respect for the complexities of each individual's body/mind. Therefore, I never want you to bypass your own judgment and what feels right while you are going through this process.

I celebrate all of you who are struggling and yet have the courage to keep going and not give up. You are my heroes. I know that within each of you is a powerful and radiant Warrioress with the strength to overcome the deep wounding you have lived through. I offer my experience, strength, support and knowledge in the hope that this process will free you from the bondage of food to be the incredible, magnificent person you are. You are now ready to begin your journey. It's time to let go and jump into this new paradigm. I'll be with you, holding your hand.

PRACTICE SESSION 2

Visual Aid: On a piece of paper, write the following key words and place them as a visual reminder in front of you. For groups, place the paper in the center of the circle. For this chapter, the sign will say:

~ The Miracle ~

(to remind you of the possibility of getting on the scale and not gaining weight)

1. Opening Attunement (see sample on p. 13 or p. 14)

If you so desire, light a candle to mark the opening of the session. I recommend that you play the subliminal *Freedom From Food* CD quietly in the background during the attunement.

2. Check-In (2–3 Minutes)

For Individuals: Write a page or more in your journal as a check-in with yourself. Next, review your homework assignments.

For Groups: Allow a 2–3-minute check-in, where you tell a little bit about yourself and share answers from the following homework assignments. (Remember to pass the talking piece and use the timer.)

• What did you observe about your feelings that came up right before you ate?

• Discuss your beliefs about food and weight that came from your observations this week.

3. 10-Minute Sharing

For Individuals: First read the following visualization and then in your journal write what comes up for you. It would be helpful at this time to read a book, such as *When Food Is Love* by Geneen Roth. It will provide stories, experiences and insights from other people who have had food problems.

For Groups: This is a special time for one person (per session) to tell a personal story. It will allow the group to get to know each other better. A lot of healing takes place by telling your story in the circle and having other people witness, support and deeply listen to you in a safe environment. Remember, you need only share what you feel comfortable talking about. To begin, the leader for the week will read the following visualization to the person whose turn it is. This will help you get in touch with what you would like to share.

Suggested Visualization to Assist the Sharing

I ask you to take a moment and close your eyes and connect with your heart. Now, I would like you to begin to follow the path that leads to your tears, pain, fear, shame, anxiety or any other emotion that connects you to your wound around food or weight (pause). Allow the important moments and events to come up (pause). Put an imaginary mirror up and look into it—not a physical look but an emotional one. What was your heart feeling then? What expression is on your face? What is your posture like? What were you needing? Tune into how you are breathing (pause). Take a moment and let any other relevant scenes or feelings arise (pause). When you are ready, slowly open your eyes. If you are in a group, share your experience.

4. Appreciations

For Individuals: This is a good time to write down three appreciations of yourself—something about your essence. See the following examples.

For Groups: Three people from the group can give brief appreciations for the person who has just spoken. An appreciation should be something about the person's essence—what you notice that stands out about that person. An appreciation should not give advice or include an explanation about how the person's story relates to your story. Here are examples of the kinds of appreciations you might offer:

I love your courage and the way you speak up for yourself.
I appreciate how you protect your Inner Child.
I think you are radiant, and I love the way you light up when you smile.

5. Break

6. Question

For Individuals: Take as long as you wish to journal about the question that follows.

For Groups: Go around the group and answer the following question. (Your timekeeper should allow each person 2 minutes to speak.)

• How does this chapter relate to your own story? How is it different?

7. Visualization Exercise

For Individuals: Read the following visualization aloud (or play the tape if you have made one). Then answer the follow-up questions.

For Groups: Choose one person to read the visualization aloud (or play the tape if someone has made one). The rest of the group members will close their eyes and sit or lie down in a comfortable position. Have your journal and a pen ready to answer the questions that follow. Then share with the group your answers. (If you run out of time, you can finish sharing next week.)

Visualization

(I recommend that you play the *FFF* subliminal CD quietly in the background.)

Find a comfortable position, sitting or lying down. I invite you to take some deep breaths. Breathe all the way in, fill all the way up with air and hold it...and then at your own pace slowly release all the air. Now, take another deep breath and hold it...and now release all the air in your body. Now, imagine that you are a tree and feel your roots going deep down into Mother Earth, grounding and relaxing you. Let them go deep into the core of her. Allow yourself, on the exhale, to release any uncomfortable feeling or tension out the bottom of your feet. Mother Earth lovingly takes it and transmutes it (pause).

Now, I would like you to imagine a big wooden door in front of you. Make it as real as you can. Note the texture, color and any details, such as the hinges, handle or knob. On the door there is a sign that says "Eater." Imagine that the part of you that has a food problem lives behind the door. Now, open the door and respectfully and sensitively allow yourself to enter her world. Just observe her. Don't get involved. Be aware of her. How does she feel? How does she look?

Now, approach her and begin to relate to her. Talk to her and listen to what she says to you…(pause). What do you want to say to her? Say it now… Allow her to respond… Give her a name that best fits her and use it when I refer to the Eater. Now, ask her to lead you back to the time in her life or a scene when she first began eating a lot and noticed she had a food problem. If you can't remember a time, make one up. Pay attention to your surroundings. Were you at home, at a friend's house, alone or with someone? Allow yourself to remember what trigger made you want to eat. Did something happen? What were you feeling right before you ate? Had someone said something to you?… or looked at you in a disturbing way?… Was there a specific interaction between yourself and someone else before you ate? Did someone touch your body in a way that was uncomfortable?… What was your mood in general at that time? What was your feeling about life then? At that time in your life, how did you feel when you woke up in the morning?…and when you went to sleep at night? Let yourself remember how you felt about yourself with friends… family… school. Did you like your body? What expression was on your face? Observe your body posture. In what areas did you have feelings of inadequacy? What word would best describe you at that time? What did you need?

Pick a few words that would generally express what you felt right before you ate. Next, picture yourself eating back then. Are you nervously eating? Is there some anxiety or emotion with which your eating is connected? Do you taste the food? Now, take a moment to review the pertinent information from this process that you want to remember. Then, slowly open your eyes and begin to answer the follow-up questions.

Follow-up Questions

(These are to be answered in silence after the visualization and then shared in the group if you are in one.)

1. The reason I began overeating was_____.

2. The scene I remember when my eating problem first began was_____.

3. By overeating, I avoid feeling_____.

4. I've generally eaten a lot in my life because _____.

5. The person (or people) who contributed the most to my eating a lot was (were)_____.

6. He or she contributed by saying_____(about me).

   By thinking_____(about me).

   By feeling_____(about me).

   By doing_____(to me).

   I generally reacted to this by_____.

8. **Homework**

   This week, your homework assignment is to do the following:

   a. Journal—What negative messages did you receive about food and weight as a child? As an adolescent? As an adult? Please list the messages and from whom they came. Describe one action step that you will do in the coming weeks to correct these messages (for example, start some form of therapy, read a book or call a nurturing friend and share what you have discovered). Once again the first step in healing these messages is to become aware of them. Do not expect them to change right away. Changing messages is a process.

   b. Inner Child Exercise—This exercise is about developing a relationship with your Inner Child. Every day, tune into your Inner Child by listening to the *FFF* CD (with audible words), where there is a section on this topic. It will assist you in dialoguing with this important part of yourself. Write down in your journal what you discover. At different times of the day, you may wish to have additional conversations with your Inner Child (for an example, see the section on Inner Child Work in How to Use This Book).

   c. (Optional) Skip ahead to the next practice session in Chapter 3 (for groups, choose one person to do this). Read Exercise 7 and, if you wish, prepare a tape in advance of the following session.

Reminder for groups: Choose a new leader for next week.

9. Appreciation

For Individuals: Write a few sentences in your journal about what most moved or inspired you in this chapter.

For Groups: Go around the circle. Speak about what most moved and inspired you in the meeting today.

10. Closing Attunement (see sample on p. 13 or p. 14)

PART II

THE FOUR MASTERY KEYS

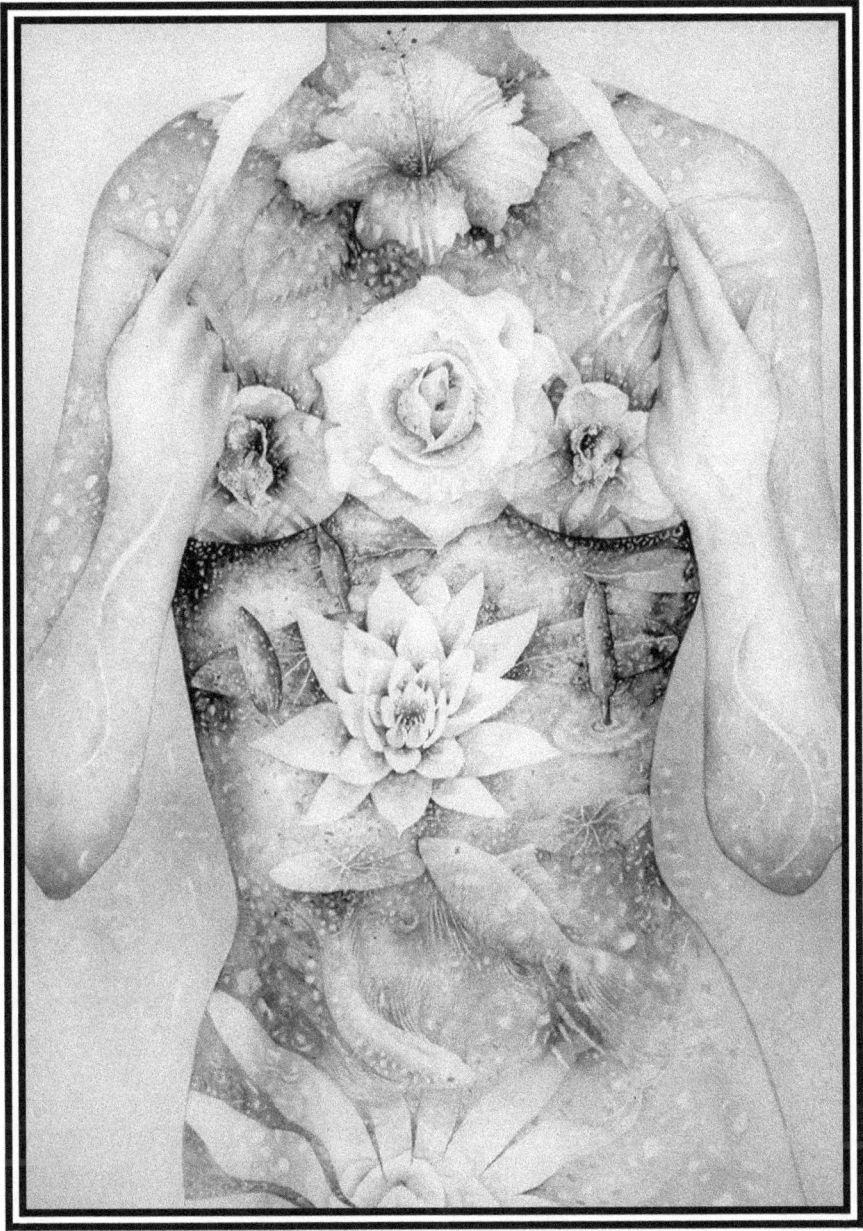

Body of Flowers by Meganne Forbes

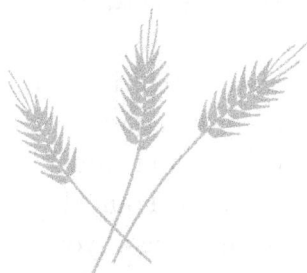

INTRODUCTION TO THE MASTERY KEYS

Part II is the entry point into the new Freedom From Food paradigm. In the next four chapters, you will learn the Mastery Keys needed to take you through the program.

To step through this gate, you must be ready to put on a new lens through which to see and focus. You are entering a world where matter is an illusion, where everything that appears solid is really fluid and constantly changing. In this place, which is truly where you live, things take form when there is a coherent, sustained vibration that coagulates around the thoughts you think.

You must come into this kingdom with the openness and the curiosity of a child, approaching these Mastery Keys from an empty place. This is required in order to understand the world that exists but is unseen. You may think you have already learned most of the ideas being presented here. At first glance, it might appear that way.

However, true, deep knowing is far beyond the intellectual. Real understanding is what affects the subatomic particles of your body, causing them to rearrange or more firmly stabilize. Therefore, to actually demonstrate these Keys, you must be able to take this new, conceptual reality and make it usable and applicable to yourself. The practice sessions at the end of each chapter are essential in assisting you through this transformation.

Part of the process is remembering and reconnecting with what actually has always existed in you. It's like the *Wizard of Oz*, when Dorothy learns she always had the power to go back home. She just had to click her feet twice, feel it in her heart and say the right words.

While repeating the phrase "There is no place like home," she is transported back. Just as Dorothy had to experience different situations with the Tin Man, Scarecrow and Lion before she could go back, so you must understand the Four Mastery Keys before you can change your body and return home to your perfect proportion.

The Tin Man did not understand that he always had a heart and the Scarecrow that he always had a brain. They had become disconnected from this knowing. It is my experience that you too must follow a path leading to the place where you can understand and demonstrate the power that has always been inside. Actually, you have always had the capability within to create the body you would like. So, let's begin creating.

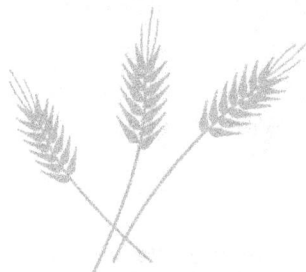

THREE

FIRST MASTERY KEY:
THE BODY HEALS ITSELF

*Homeostasis is the ability of an organism to respond appropriately
to any given circumstance, and then return to a base line of what
would be called normal functioning.*

—Peter Levine, PhD

Meeting the Wise Woman

You are now entering the first step of your journey. Allow your-self to take a deep breath and become centered. As you stand at the threshold of this new paradigm about food and weight, open the doors and windows that house your magnificent imagination. Picture your old, outmoded ideas as a cloak that you take off and leave behind. Allow it to fall away as you visualize yourself walking through a beautiful lush forest on sacred land. Enliven your senses as you take in the clean earthy smells, ancient old trees, dancing creeks and the hum of insects and animals. Slowly advancing toward you is a Wise Woman, who with a strong, grounded presence will be your guide on this journey. She stands in front of you, gazing into your eyes until a feeling of safety and comfort opens between you.

Taking you by the hand, she leads you to a very unusual place, where you will learn and absorb new information. When you arrive, she invites you to sit across from her in a comfortable chair made of all-natural fibers. She asks that you close your eyes and deeply attune

49

to the magical healing sounds of nature. As you resonate with your surroundings, the Wise Woman begins to speak:

—⁓—

I call upon you to move into the vast universe of your mind, expanding into some new ideas and truths about your body. Already encoded at birth is your ideal weight and proportion. The basic blueprint of this design is one of self-healing, and with rare exceptions, it is exquisitely perfect and unchanging. Although extra pounds might veil what is truly there, your physical perfection does exist within. I want you to welcome in the idea that a healthy body is your birthright.

For the next while, you will study and activate *the inner workings and natural flow of your physical form.* You will become aware of how your body was set up from the formless to orchestrate and maintain precisely your ideal proportion—a creative masterpiece. What you will learn now, which may surprise you, is that *your body is actually your friend in the battle against weight.*

As you access the ways your physical form balances and repairs itself, you will begin to understand the miracle of the *First Mastery Key—the Body Heals Itself (and Is Designed to Maintain Its Perfect Proportion).*

—⁓—

Now, bringing your awareness back, you are ready to explore this first new Key. You will meet this Wise Woman throughout the book at the beginning of each chapter to introduce the new FFF ideas and support you on your way in this transformational process.

The Body Heals Itself Automatically

Our body parts do their jobs as diligently as ants on an anthill, carrying out a mission to build and sustain their environment. I remember learning about the body's amazing ability to heal *automatically* when I was a small child. One day, I fell down and scraped my knee. Seeing blood on my knee was scary. I wasn't sure what it meant or what would happen to me. However, soon I learned that no matter how often I fell down and scraped my knee, my body would somehow take care of itself. It would *dependably* send out white blood cells to kill the bacteria. My blood would clot, and my skin would form a scab. Then the scab would go away. No matter how many times I fell down, my body always healed itself like clockwork in an eloquent dance of health.

This is the miracle, the wondrous way the body mends even when we don't do a thing! I did not have to say affirmations ("My knee is now healing. My knee is now healing."). I wasn't even old enough to understand what an affirmation was. I discovered that *I could count on my body*—whether I was awake or asleep—to heal all wounds.

I trusted my body and its self-governing system more as a child than as an adult. Part of my growth process was reconnecting with the automatic healing mechanism inherent in my physical form. I knew that being overweight was not a healthy state. I thought I needed to diet or do something outside of myself. *What I did not know was that my body itself was trying to help rid me of my extra pounds.*

How Your Body Is Organized

Imagine yourself shrinking down, small enough to sit on the sidelines inside your physical form. See the multitude of incredibly intricate and complex systems working as a team. Watch how highly organized and intelligent they are. The blood is circulating through rivers of veins and arteries, your heart is keeping a constant beat, air is coming in and going out, and on and on.

Overall, a force that is constantly self-organizing toward the highest level of health guides this process. Since your optimum weight is part of your health, it is the place to which your body will try to return. *Your body ceaselessly tries to eliminate anything you ingest that is unneeded or toxic—whether it is excess weight or food.* You actually have to go against this force to put on extra pounds. It is easy to feel victimized by a never-ending battle with the scale, forgetting that you have ongoing help 24/7. This help is like a constant gravitational pull back to your ideal form. Pause here for a moment, closing your eyes and visualizing this intricate system of intelligence at work.

Hippocrates said, "The natural healing force within us is the greatest force in getting well." People who are thin (meaning in their perfect proportion) rely on this pull in the body to always maintain ideal weight. They never question it. They have a knowing that unneeded food will move right through them and not add extra pounds—and it does.

Allow yourself to imagine this happening in your own body. Take a moment and mentally zoom inside. Visualize yourself eating a cookie. Then picture an inner team that immediately takes the cookie and begins to break it down. The team takes from the food what your body needs and eliminates the rest. See your body as a unified organism, efficient and precise, moving the food directly into various organs and the digestive system. Without interference, watch how your food is transformed rather smoothly until all excess is eliminated. In the next months as you begin to understand and follow the FFF principles, you can count on this force *and be able to relax more when you are eating.*

Learning to Trust

Sometimes people ask me, "What do you do if you are full because you ate too much? Don't you worry about gaining weight and getting fat? Don't you worry that you are heavier?" My answer is, "No"! I trust my body. If I am full, the feeling may go away in an hour, or it may take overnight. However, my body *always* handles it.

I trust my body to do its *natural job of elimination and bring me back to a state of equilibrium and balance.* If this weren't true, I would blow up like a hot air balloon and explode. Let yourself remember a time when you got stuffed on pancakes or at a holiday meal. Within the next day or so, you did not feel stuffed anymore. The full feeling went away. That's because your body eliminated the excess. Remember, *full does not equal fat!!!* I do not try to second-guess how my body does this. Nor do I interfere by imposing on it my own ideas of dieting, exercise or fasting.

Your body is your holy temple. It houses your precious being. It was created perfectly and knows what to do. When you can completely internalize and accept this fact, you will gain a new level of confidence. This confidence is one of the secrets to success in this program.

When people say, "Patricia, what happens when you look in the mirror and see a roll around your waist and it seems like you've gained weight?" I tell them that I go into trust. I trust my body to work for me. I trust that this is a temporary state of fluctuation and that my body will return to a state of balanced proportion. It will eliminate whatever is not supposed to be there, and it always does. I have *absolute confidence* in my body.

By the way, I say the same thing if I am bloated from eating salt or from my menstrual cycle. In a normally functioning person, this is a *temporary state*. You can trust your physical form to *self-regulate*. What can you say to yourself if you are bloated for any reason? *"Bloat Does Not Equal Weight!!!"*

I am not proposing that it is good to eat until you are full or to ignore the fact that it doesn't feel good when you eat too much. What I *am* saying is that being full or bloated will not affect your weight, that you can *trust your body* to eliminate excess. Do you hear the distinction? Your body will respond to the subtleties of what you believe and say to yourself.

What About Exercise?

This may surprise you, but in my opinion, how much you weigh is not necessarily connected to the amount that you exercise. We have been encouraged to think that we have to exercise to lose weight. I have had aerobic instructors and body builders in my program who were afraid to stop working out because they were sure they would gain extra pounds. Some of them were taking or teaching three to four exercise classes a day! When people willfully use physical activity in this way, they are sometimes thought of as "exercise bulimics." I quote one of the participants, Barbara, who said, "I trained for a marathon by running many miles a day, and I never lost a pound." Another participant, Cathy, also said she trained for a marathon. She reported running 20–25 miles a week for 7 months and never lost weight.

In my experience with myself and with my groups, I have found that *you do not have to exercise to stay at your optimum weight or get thin.* Many times in my life I did very little exercise—sometimes nothing at all for weeks, sometimes only several 45-minute strolls on the beach—*and I did not put on extra pounds.* I recommend that avid exercisers work out minimally during the 2-Week Healing process (Chapter 9) to prove this to themselves. This allows you to disconnect from the concept of working out to lose weight. If you depend on activities to maintain your perfect proportion, then what would happen if you were sick, injured, bedridden or hospitalized?

Don't get me wrong. I believe exercise is an essential component for body/mind/spirit balance. I am not telling you to avoid working out or that it is not good for you. It is something you can do for a better quality of life, for being toned and for mental clarity. What I am discouraging here is the mental association between exercise and losing or maintaining weight. *I now do physical activities because they make me feel good* and help reduce stress.

Note: At this point, you might be saying, "I hear what you're telling me, but I still don't feel I can trust my body." That is perfectly normal. There is much to learn in the next months before you can rest in that knowing. The following sections will help you create more trust. Layer upon layer, you will build a foundation that is strong enough to uphold this new weight paradigm.

Homeostasis

Homeostasis is one of the functions within the body that keeps it healthy and at your optimum weight. Through this process, *your physical form is always balancing the input of fluctuations* from inner and outer environments. Homeostasis creates equilibrium in your system. For example, the body balances itself as it actively regulates temperature from 98.6 to 98.7 degrees Fahrenheit. Equilibrium is present in blood glucose and water levels as well.

In regard to weight, homeostasis governs your body's perfect proportion by *taking the nourishment it needs from what you ingest and discarding the rest.* When I was a child, there was so little awareness of health food in general and none in my family. I was raised on white bread, which we would first roll into dough balls. It was mostly air. We also devoured cookies, potato chips, candy, ice cream—you name it, we ate it. I didn't think about diets or even know what they were until high school, but my body always found balance. I was thin in those early years. I never thought to question how my body was eliminating the food I consumed.

To be at your optimum weight, *do you have to know how your body does this? No. Do you have to see how it does this? No.* (Some people ask if I go to the bathroom more on this program. The answer is "No.") You do not need to comprehend the details of how things are expelled from the body. You just need to *allow and trust* it to do its job.

Your Elimination System

The body keeps healthy and at its optimum weight through an intricate elimination system that expels toxins and unneeded waste. Your skin is your biggest elimination organ. It constantly removes excess energy through the pores when you perspire, get a rash and so on. Your kidneys and liver also act as filters. The liver creates bile, which breaks down food during digestion, while your kidneys separate waste products and water from the blood. A great deal is distilled through your hair as well. According to Gay Hendricks in his book *Conscious Breathing,* up to 70 percent of the toxins in your body are released through yet another method—your breath.

Try visualizing excess food moving off of you like steam leaving a teapot (pause). Your physical form is always trying to purify itself in a continuous flow toward optimal health.

The Perfect Proportion Within

It is important to have a set point in your mind as to where your body is trying to return. For this reason, we will explore the perfect proportion that lives inside you and all other living things. By observing the things in nature with which humans have not tampered, you can attune yourself to the ideal size within.

First, understand that fat is a manmade idea. It does not exist in nature. Ask yourself, "Are there any fat or thin trees?" Let yourself picture some trees or go look at them. They may have different types of bark, and their shapes, curves and sizes may be different. However, it is easy to see that all of them are perfectly proportioned. Even though there are numerous kinds of trees with various tree trunks, you would never refer to any of them as "fat" or "thin." You can see how silly this identification would be when applied to nature. Also, it is important to note that trees take in food all day long from the sun and the soil. *They never diet. They absorb what they need and release the rest.* You will find the same truths apparent in flowers. Allow yourself to observe several varieties. Experience the different colors, shapes, sizes and smells. You would never think, "Oh, what a heavy flower!" or "Doesn't that flower look anorexic!" They are just flowers with perfectly proportioned petals and stems.

Next, think of several animals in the wild—a sleek deer, a bird, a monkey. Think of the insects, fish and reptiles. They all have a "just right" look—not fat, not thin.

Fat manifests in nature only in situations that have been tampered with by man. For example, fixing a dog often makes it gain weight. Domesticating animals, putting them in cages or restricting their diet can also result in extra pounds. These are human interventions. *Never in a healthy, natural environment do you see fat animals.* Take time to identify with the perfection that exists in the natural world.

Nature is powerful. It is fully capable of maintaining its perfection. When there is too much water, there are floods. When the clouds are too heavy, it rains. When forests are too full, fires break out. You are a part of this macrocosm and have similar, natural balancing processes within you.

The image of what perfect proportion looks like exists within you right now. Take a moment to pause and feel this. If you can't do this yet, *just make it up. This sets the energy in motion* (that is, fake it 'til you make it). Your optimum weight may be covered over by all kinds of (mental) illusion, but nevertheless it is there—like the sun, which always comes out after dark clouds pass by. As you peel away all layers of illusion, you will find the essential you in your perfect body weight still shining.

In Conclusion

Without a doubt, *your body always works to heal itself and return to its perfect proportion.* Right now, inside you exists an ideal form—one that is unique and "just right" for you. This natural state is unlike media images of overly thin models and liposuctioned movie stars. The FFF program *will not* take you to an unnatural weight that is less than your optimum proportion.

Hopefully, you are embracing the idea that your body can heal itself and that it is your ally in this quest to lose excess pounds. Your body is not an enemy, but your friend. The secret is learning to *trust it.*

PRACTICE SESSION 3

Note: It may take 2 weeks to complete the exercises in this session. Each week, repeat steps 1–4 and then continue where you left off with the exercises. Always end with the final appreciations and closing attunement.

Visual Aid: On a piece of paper, write the following key words and place them as a visual reminder in front of you. For groups, place this paper in the center of the circle. For this chapter, the sign will say:

~ *The Body Heals Itself* ~
(and is designed to maintain its perfect proportion)

1. Opening Attunement (see sample on p. 13 or p. 14)

If you so desire, light a candle to mark the opening of the session. I recommend that you play the subliminal *Freedom From Food* CD quietly in the background during the attunement.

2. Check–In (2–3 Minutes)

For Individuals: Write a page or more in your journal, checking in with yourself and reviewing your homework from the previous chapter.

For Groups: Allow a 2–3-minute check-in for each person. Tell a little bit about how you are doing with the program and what you discovered from the following homework question. If something else more pressing is going on in your life, please also speak about that. (Remember to pass the talking piece and use the timer.)

- What negative messages did you receive about food and weight as a child? As an adolescent? As an adult? Describe one thing that you will do in the coming weeks to correct these messages (for example, get massage or other bodywork, therapy, read a book, call a nurturing friend).

3. 10-Minute Sharing

For Individuals: First read the following visualization and then

58

write in your journal what comes up for you. In addition, you may want to read a book (such as *When Food Is Love*, by Geneen Roth) for these 10 minutes to learn about other people's stories.

For Groups: This is a special time for one person (per session) to tell a personal story. It will allow you to get to know each other better. A lot of healing takes place by telling your story into the circle and having other people witness, support and deeply listen to you in a safe environment. Remember, you need only share what you feel comfortable talking about. To begin, the leader can read the following visualization to the person whose turn it is. This will help you get in touch with what you would like to share.

Suggested Visualization to Assist the Sharing

I ask you to take a moment and close your eyes and connect with your heart. Now, I would like you to begin to follow the path that leads to your tears, pain, fear, shame, anxiety or any other emotion that connects you to your wound around food or weight (pause). Allow the important moments and events to come up (pause). Put an imaginary mirror up and look into it—not a physical look but an emotional one. What was your heart feeling then? What were you needing? What expression is on your face? What is your posture like? Tune into how you are breathing (pause). Take a moment and let any other relevant scenes or feelings arise (pause). When you are ready, slowly open your eyes. If you are in a group, share your experience.

4. Appreciations

For Individuals: This is a good time to write down three appreciations of yourself—something about your essence. See the examples that follow.

For Groups: Three people from the group can give brief appreciations for the person who has just spoken. An appreciation should be something about one's essence—what you notice that stands out about that person. An appreciation should not give advice or include an explanation about how the person's story relates to your story. Here are some examples of the kinds of appreciations you might offer:

I love your courage and the way you speak up for yourself.
I appreciate how you protect your Inner Child.
I think you are radiant, and I love the warmth and welcome that you offer to everyone.

5. Break

6. Discussion

For Individuals: In your journal, write responses to the following topics.

For Groups: Go around the circle and talk about the following topics. (Remember to pass the talking piece and use a timer.)

- Share any new thoughts or feelings that surfaced after reading this chapter about trusting your body.

- Share a personal example of a time when you saw that your body or someone else's body healed itself. For example, it may be a time when you got sick and your body repaired itself quickly.

- Share an example of a time in your life when you were able to eat whatever you wanted, your body eliminated what you didn't need automatically and you didn't gain any weight (think of times when you were younger, holidays, vacations, being in love, etc.).

- Review the meaning of homeostasis and how this process helps you manage your weight.

7. Visualization Exercise

For Individuals: Read the following visualization aloud (or play the tape if you have made one). Then answer the questions that follow.

For Groups: Choose one person to read the visualization aloud (or play the tape if someone has made one). The rest of the group members will close their eyes and sit or lie down in a comfortable position. Have your journal and a pen ready to answer the questions that follow. Then share with the group your answers.

Visualization

*I invite you to find a comfortable position and begin to allow your-
self to relax. Close your eyes and take three deep breaths. Now, let your
imagination carry you back to when you first remember overeating
(pause). Focus on the part of yourself that you named the Eater in the
visualization from the last session. Allow yourself to reexperience the feelings and emotions you felt when you first began eating a lot. Bring back
the memory in your body/mind whether you were feeling mad, sad, glad,
angry, anxious or scared.*

*See if there was anyone you trusted and felt safe to talk to at the time.
Was there someone who would have loved you and respected your feelings? Did anyone really know who you were inside? Did anyone know
what your heart was feeling? Did anyone realize what you were needing
or how you felt about yourself? Was there anyone who was interested?*

*Now, see all of the important people at that time in a circle around
you (your family, friends, etc.). Observe, one by one, their facial expres-
sions, tones of voices, words and looks. If you had told these people about
the emotional pain you were in, what do you think would have happened? Fantasize the whole scene now. Maybe you did tell them and got
blasted. Maybe you felt too much shame or embarrassment to tell them,
or too much pride, or maybe it was fear. Whatever it was that caused you
to hold back, observe that now (pause).*

*Next, let yourself see how intelligent you were to have eaten your feel-
ings away rather than to have shared them with people who might have
been uncaring and abusive. Give yourself a lot of love for protecting yourself, your feelings and your heart in order to survive.*

*Get in touch with how you covered up these feelings so that people
around you wouldn't know them. How did you shield yourself from outside pain and from fearful, threatening and devaluing circumstances?
Did you put on a tough persona, acting like you had it together when you
were really scared and unsure of yourself? Were you helpful and a "good
girl," so they would think everything was just fine with you? Were you a
people pleaser? Did you sulk and mope and not let them near you? Did
you act angry and rebel and not let them know how fragile, scared and*

hurt you were inside?

Whatever role you played so they wouldn't see your pain, remind yourself of it now and watch yourself reenacting it (pause). Observe yourself carefully. How does your body feel while you are doing this? How does your heart feel?

Now, put your Inner Child on the lap of your Nurturing Adult and hold her in the perfect way that feels good to her. If she would like it, hug her and stroke her hair. Reassure her that she is no longer in that uncomfortable situation and that now there are safe people around (especially her Loving Adult). They can listen to her and love her. Take a moment and allow your Nurturing Adult to give her exactly what she is needing right now.

Next, gently and slowly allow yourself to start to come back into the room or environment in which you began. Feel your body begin to move. Gently open your eyes. Ground yourself by breathing the energy up from the core of Mother Earth through your feet. Remain in silence as you answer the follow-up questions.

a. The most important people around me at that time were
_____.

b. The main reasons I did not share my feelings with them were
_____.

c. The role I played so that they would not know my true feelings was
_____.

d. The way I hide my insecurities from people now is_____.

e. I think people would describe me as_____.

f. The way that this differs from who I am inside or how I really feel inside is_____.

g. Today, the following people know how out of control I am at certain times _____.

h. The places where I feel competent in my life are _____.

i. Do the people who see your competence know the extent of your pain and hurt inside?_____.

j. Are you afraid to express your needs or ask for help from others?
_____.

*k. What did you learn about people in your family who leaned on others or who showed signs of weakness?*_____.

8. Exercise in Nature (See also the section called The Perfect Proportion Within in this chapter.)

For this exercise, you will need to go to a place that has trees, flowers, birds and other animals, if possible.

To begin, find a comfortable place to sit in silence. You may have to move to different viewing spots during the exercise. Bring your journal. Start by reading the following paragraphs as you make observations about your surroundings.

Our bodies are always trying to heal, and nature shows us the state to which our bodies are trying to return. We can look to nature for various examples of what appears as perfect proportion.

As you observe different things in this natural setting, make a mental picture of what perfect proportion feels like and looks like. Experience it in your body. To start, take a moment and focus on the wild animals and insects around you (pause). You would never say, "Oh that's a fat bird," or, "What a thin butterfly," or, "That ant is too thin." All animals and insects that live in the wild have a just right look. They always are in their perfect proportion. They are not too fat or too thin. Imagine what it feels like to be in their bodies (pause).

Creatures in the wild never worry about dieting or taking in too much food. As if you had a camera in your forehead, snap a picture of them to keep the memory of perfect proportion alive in your mind so that you can refer to it when needed.

Humans have made themselves feel separate, but there is no separation between nature and yourself. Know the truth about the perfect proportion that exists in all things and in yourself as you look at the trees around you. Some trees have bigger trunks, but they are perfect. You would never say, "That tree trunk is too fat," because it is perfectly proportioned for its size. Each tree has its own size and shape.

Begin opening to your own perfect proportion—not too fat, not too thin, where you just "are." Begin to feel what it feels like to be "just right." Get a sense of it. Know it. Take a deep breath in and imagine it. Let the trees trigger that sense of a natural proportion to which your body is trying to return. Keep this picture in your mind as a reminder (take a long pause as you rest your eyes on different trees).

Now, I would like you to observe some flowers. Notice not only the flower itself but also each petal that is perfectly proportioned. Know that the same law of proportion that applies to flowers applies to you. You would never say, "Oh, there's a fat flower or a thin flower." It's just a flower. Fat is a manmade idea and manifestation that is unnatural (pause and observe several kinds of flowers).

Next, observe some leaves. These leaves can act as a catalyst to remind you of your optimum proportion. Each leaf is the perfect size—not too fat, not too thin. There are no anorexic or bulimic leaves. Notice also the orderliness of their design.

Now, I would like you to think of some young children. In general, children are perfectly proportioned, unless they have received some early programming or have a medical condition. Even if they consume sweets and junk food, their perfect proportion is still naturally maintained. Can you recall some children you know who eat like this and remain thin? Do you remember a time when you ate lots of junk food, like they do, and you kept your natural proportion (pause)? If so, feel that feeling again now. If not, create the feeling with your imagination.

As a part of nature, we have a perfectly proportioned state that is a reflection of our being. Know that nature is powerful. It wants to maintain balance (in a similar way that homeostasis balances our bodies). When there is too much water, there are floods. When the clouds are too heavy, it rains. When forests are too full, there are fires. Nature is always trying to return to a balanced, proportioned state. As part of nature, our bodies also are trying to maintain perfection. They are working with every breath we take to keep us healthy and at our optimum weight by eliminating all that is unhealthy, excess or toxic.

Now, take a few moments and allow yourself to digest the parts of this exercise that had the greatest impact on you. Keep all of the wonderful images in your head while you continue working through this program. Now, take some time to write your thoughts in your journal.

For Groups: Take 3–5 minutes to share in the circle what you wrote. (Don't forget to use the talking piece and the timer.)

8. Homework

This week, your homework assignment is to do the following:

a. Inner Child Exercise—Continue developing your relationship with your Inner Child daily by listening to the *Freedom From Food* CD with spoken words. Write in your journal what you discover.

b. Journal—Write any thoughts you have this week about how the body heals itself, or about the idea of perfect proportion that exists in all natural things.

c. Answer the Question—To prepare for this FFF healing, what can you do to strengthen your connection to your Higher Self or Spirit? What steps will you take? For example, you can learn to meditate, read inspiring books, learn more about your Adult Self so you can nurture your Inner Child and so on.

d. Statements of Trust—Throughout this program, your ability to *trust* your physical organism will grow stronger. Keep the following paragraph where you can see it daily in order to build a more powerful relationship with your body.

*I totally **trust** my body to heal itself.*

I never waiver.

*If I am full, I **trust** my body to eliminate all unnecessary food.*

I never think what I eat will make me gain weight.

I know my body naturally maintains its perfect proportions.

*I deeply and completely **trust** my body to eliminate and maintain my ideal weight.*

*If I am bloated, I **trust** my body to remove the bloat.*

I know full does not equal fat.
I know bloat does not equal weight.
*I **trust** my body to eliminate it.*
*I **trust** my body.*

Reminder for groups: Choose a new leader for next week.

9. Appreciation

For Individuals: Write a few sentences in your journal about what most moved or inspired you in this chapter.

For Groups: Go around the circle. Speak about what most moved and inspired you in the meeting today.

10. Closing Attunement (see sample on p. 13 or p. 14)

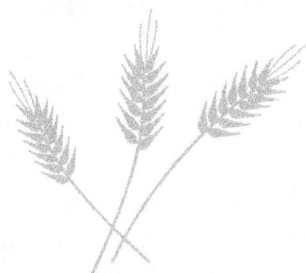

FOUR

SECOND MASTERY KEY: MIND CREATES MATTER

Body and mind are one.... The body is the actual outward manifestation, in physical space, of the mind.

—Candace B. Pert, PhD, *Molecules of Emotion*

Mind is the matrix of all matter.

—Max Planck, physicist and Nobel Prize winner, quoted by Gregg Braden in *The Isaiah Effect*

The Wise Woman Speaks

You have now investigated the perfection that is inherent in the body system and all of nature. You have viewed the same principles in the trees, the flowers, the animals and your own body. You have come to understand that you are a part of nature.

It is now important to ask yourself, *"What has caused my weight problem? What has gone wrong?"* You are aware that your body is always trying to heal itself and that a homeostatic process inherent in your body is always working to balance your weight. Therefore, why are you not in your perfect body? What is the difference between you and those beautifully proportioned animals you have been observing?

The answer is in *Mastery Key Two—Mind Creates Matter.* The difference between you and the animals is your ability to cocreate with your thoughts, emotions and beliefs. They are the catalysts that tell your cells where to go and that create the bridge to get there. They act as attractors, rearranging your physical form. As magnetizers, they draw your body away from perfect proportion or back to it. The secret to changing your body does not lie in a special diet, rigorous exercise or magic supplements. It lies in the power of your own mind.

The Body/Mind Connection

According to quantum physics, nature (including your body) is affected at the subatomic level by your participation. Scientists have documented that the presence of an observer affects the motion of the tiny, nanoparticles of matter. If the observer expects them to behave in a certain way, they will. Studies have shown that at the moment of observation by a conscious mind, the electron chooses what it will do based on the observer's expectations.

Scientist David Albert, author of *Quantum Mechanics and Experience,* concurs that our conscious minds direct the actions of these particles, changing the universe from a vague collection of possibilities into the more definite reality that we know. Our conscious choices allow the universe to select what it will be, how it will appear and how it will behave.

In his book *The Isaiah Effect,* scientist Gregg Braden remarks that the choices we make take place in a field of energy that exists in every aspect of creation. This field has intelligence that responds to emotions and thoughts. In the FFF program, we are looking at our body's weight as part of this creation. We deduce that, at the subatomic level, our bodies are also directly influenced by our thinking and emotions and will always meet our expectations.

In the case of food, for example, you might believe that bread and butter make you gain weight. Take a moment to imagine what happens as a result of this belief. It logically follows that your body will be reorganizing around this expectation. Rather than releasing unneeded energy automatically, your body will begin to hold onto it. The atoms coalesce around the cognition, creating an obstruction that interferes with your body's natural elimination process. It is like being at the ocean, getting an idea to build a sand castle and then taking thousands of tiny grains of sand and creating that form. This is what your mind does with your deliberations.

Your consciousness is most likely bombarded with countless thoughts about food, both self-imposed and from the outside world. Your mind is constantly accepting and rejecting one concept after another. "Don't eat this. It has too many calories. Don't eat that. It has too many carbohydrates or too much fat." These messages create mistrust. "Your body can't handle this food," they say. "You are going to get fat." Words and fears from the outside seep into your mind and bombard your perfectly ordered inner ecosystem. Instead of a clear, flowing stream, your thoughts become a dam of confusion, causing your body to hold onto food that it would otherwise eliminate effortlessly.

Remember, your mind and emotions direct the energy from which your body is created. Are you thinking like Teflon or like Velcro? Are you letting excess food energy slide off your nonstick surface, or are you holding onto it like you'll never let go?

The Power of Your Conscious Mind

The good news is that you have the power to choose consciously which thoughts you put into your mind and which ones you focus on. One important way you create in your world is through your psyche. A sculptor first gets an idea of what she wants to create and then creates it. An architect first thinks out the plans for a house before it is built. Therefore, take a moment and imagine the body you would like to live in.

In a sense, *your thoughts are prophetic*. They become alive and vibrate throughout your body. Whatever you think becomes a preview of what manifests in the physical realm. Since your thoughts can rearrange matter, it is important to choose your words carefully and set targets that anchor what you wish to manifest.

Because your body acquiesces to your every wish, rearranging your living organism as you speak, you need to develop an awareness of how thoughts affect weight. If you say to yourself, "I just look at those chocolate chip cookies and gain weight," guess what? You set that possibility in motion. Beliefs are so strong that some people gain weight eating grapefruit and lettuce. *If you think a certain food will make you fat, it will.*

Using Thoughts to Affect Your Body

Biofeedback researchers have found that by changing your thoughts, you can directly change your bodily symptoms. During a biofeedback session, you are connected to a machine that monitors your physical responses. You are then asked to concentrate on phrases or visualizations for the purpose of changing your physiological state. Often these words and images are designed to create states of relaxation and confidence. The technique is used to alleviate headaches, high blood pressure, migraines, anxiety and many other problems.

Gregg Braden also talks about how one's thoughts and feelings can affect the body. In *The Isaiah Effect*, he writes about a group of people who worked on a patient who was later healed of a tumor. The problem corrected when the people concentrated their thoughts and feelings on the ideas that the tumor had never existed, the patient was perfectly healthy and the body was already healed.

> *Their actions became the attractor for a choice point, allowing the quantum leap from a course of events already under way, to a new course with a different outcome.... Contrary to the suggestion that such change occurs slowly, over long periods, the new possibility was brought into focus, and the original released, in two minutes and forty seconds!*

Masura Emoto, a doctor of alternative medicine, has done extensive research on a related subject: the connection between consciousness and water. Since our bodies are 70 percent water, his research is essential to understanding how our mental activity affects our weight. Emoto studied how water responds to words. His findings show that water crystals became distorted and imploded when confronted with negative words, such as "You make me sick." However, words such as *love* and *gratitude* produced beautiful water crystal patterns.

In the book *Messages From Water*, Emoto observed that

...the elementary particle that is found in atoms has no regularity in modern science. The reason is that it changes according to the consciousness of observers by the way they see things. The world of the neutrino is at the same consciousness level as that of human beings. That is why the root level of matter depends on people's consciousness.

Right now, let yourself pause and say some kind words to your body. Feel the way it responds. Try saying, "Everything I eat makes me lighter and lighter," and see how it feels. Remember, *whenever you direct your focus, energy starts moving* toward that reality.

When I was a young child, my mother used to tell me that I had a lucky star. She also told me that as a baby, I was called "Smiling Island" because I was so happy. These wonderful, powerful messages were given to me at the essential level before my problems began. I have carried those thoughts with me all of my life. They are like a loving balm to my soul that reassures me when life gets challenging. Whenever I bring those thoughts to mind, they uplift my frequency and renew the water crystals that make up my body.

In *The Only Diet There Is*, well-known author and workshop leader Sondra Ray said, "The thoughts you have about food are what make it fattening." She reported that a study done on people at their desired weight showed they all had *one thought in common*: "... they could eat whatever and whenever they wanted without gaining weight." This is *just one seemingly small thought, yet it is part of the glue* that keeps slender people at their ideal weight.

I say the same thing when people ask me how I can eat so much and stay so thin. I simply know that I never gain weight from food. I invite you to visit this reality and begin to think like this.

The Unconscious Mind

Unconscious thoughts are just as critical to investigate as the ones in your awareness. These veiled thoughts can affect your well-being without your knowledge. It can often take professional help to track them and begin the healing process. For example, you may wonder why you always think that you are not intelligent enough or pretty enough but can't recall the incident that makes you feel this way.

People are continually receiving these kinds of messages from the collective consciousness of our society. Popular stereotypes override reality and affect us all the time. For example, mass beliefs beckon us to go on diets in order to look like skinny models. We can find ourselves acting like robots, reshaping ourselves to current fads and sexy fashions in the hope that they will get us the love we are missing. It is no accident that cosmetic surgery is such a craze. We are driven by externalizations, so desperate for acceptance that on a deep level we disconnect from our authentic selves. Unfortunately, we are not aware of how much we have been influenced by outside programming.

Your subconscious mind works like a computer. It records the input without modification, reflecting your thoughts without addition or subtraction. If you type in "Carbohydrates make me fat," your subconscious mind registers that exact information. It doesn't add something, such as "If I eat them before 6 o'clock, it's OK." Therefore, be careful to say what you mean. The information you choose to listen to and believe will program your subconscious mind.

Your body is also the record keeper of the deep, unconscious emotional wounds that were too much for your psyche to bear. They might have been horrific things that happened to you personally or perhaps things you observed. They got buried for your protection, so you would not fragment and fall to pieces from overwhelming pain. Tucked away yet unresolved, they are sometimes inviolable secrets even to you. However, they are still alive and influencing you. Like parasites, they are feeding off your energy and must be brought up to the surface for release. You might get a sneak preview of these deep feelings in your dreams. Allow them to reveal the locked, secret places that imprison you.

Negative parental messages also go directly into a young child's unconscious. Unfortunately, many children have been told that they will never amount to anything and that they are defective and inadequate in various ways. These beliefs can plague people for a lifetime and stop them from manifesting what they want in life.

People often try to tell themselves it is safe to be thin while their unconscious mind contradicts them by saying they don't deserve it. When this is cleared up and your emotions and thoughts are aligned with an intention, manifestation becomes possible. For this deep work, I recommend methods such as Eye Movement Desensitization and Reprocessing (EMDR), the Emotional Freedom Technique (EFT, see Chapter 7 in the section Tap Your Saboteurs Away), hypnosis or psychotherapy.

Motivational Tapes and Visualization

The unconscious mind can be a powerful, constructive resource if it is used deliberately to create positive outcomes. This is the reason why so many athletes and business moguls use motivational tapes to program themselves for success. They know that accessing the unconscious part of the psyche can increase their skills.

In addition to motivational tapes, visualization is a powerful way to use the unconscious. College sports teams, pro athletes and the U.S. Olympic Committee have sports psychologists who train athletes to visualize positive images for peak performance. I read in *U.S.A. Weekend* (1994) that gold medal swimmer Janet Evans pictures every stroke she is about to take. Think about it. Who has a better chance of winning? The woman who tells herself, "I know I won't make it. I always fail," or the woman who pictures in her mind, "I can do it. I've got what it takes!"

In extreme situations, a powerful image can even help people exceed their physical capabilities. Give people a cause to which they can dedicate their actions, such as a dying parent or a god to believe in, and they will go the extra mile even with no more fight left. Every time they recall the picture or thought of their purpose, a surge of energy catapults them beyond what the mind thinks it can ordinarily do. Using the visualizations and exercises in this program, you can tap into this same power to change your relationship with food and weight.

In the book *Getting Well Again*, Dr. Carl Simonton pioneered using visualization techniques to assist his cancer patients. Some of them were able to enlist the power of their minds to reduce cancerous masses. In his findings, he concluded that patients' participation in their own healing was extremely important.

In one experiment, he chose two groups of people with bleeding ulcers. Both groups were given placebos. People in the first group were told that this pill would absolutely make them better. Those in the second group were told that the effect would be uncertain. The study showed that 75 percent of the first group got better compared with only 25 percent of the second group—a powerful demonstration of the body/mind connection.

Shapeshifting

One of the exciting discoveries of the *Freedom From Food* program is that when your thoughts are aligned with the principles, you can actually change your body weight in a very short time—a few days, a few hours or even a few minutes! I refer to this as a kind of shapeshifting, which is possible when intention and conviction are strongly present. Here are some actual examples from FFF participants to demonstrate the astounding possibilities of your body/mind. (**Note:** These individuals had completed the 2-Week Healing in Chapter 9 and proven to themselves the unlimited power of their own thinking.)

~

It was during a weekend where there was to be a family gathering—and my Warrioress was ready to face them all! Prior to pack-

ing for the trip, I had tried on my outfit to see how coordinated it looked. Part of it included a loose-fitting skirt. The morning of the event, I could feel some of that old, tired, low self-esteem sneaking in, and sure enough, as I put on my skirt, I could barely zip it up. But my Warrioress was not going to let anyone get the best of me. I went into the restroom and stood before the mirror and reassured myself of my newfound beliefs: "My Higher Self is protecting me. I am beautiful and thin. I am a radiant child of light, and it is safe to let myself shine!" I then trusted that I would be OK. Within a matter of 10 minutes, as I was adjusting myself one last time in the mirror, my skirt was suddenly inches looser! It is truly amazing how powerful our minds are, and when they are used properly, our sabotaging thoughts don't stand a chance!

—Participant

There have been many times in my life when I felt the actual size of my body shift dramatically from the time I got dressed in the morning until the evening, making my clothes incredibly uncomfortable. I remember thinking, "What is this about? Do I have a digestion problem? Is it gas?" It seemed unexplainable! Knowing my body was healthy, I just accepted it as what my body did.

Well into the Freedom From Food program, I experienced a situation at work where I was feeling "less than" another person. Throughout a 3-day job, I had been giving my power away to her. This seemed to simultaneously slow down the way my body processed food. I got larger and larger until, by the end of the last day, I could not even zip up the pants that I comfortably had put on in the morning.

I called Patricia the next day, freaking out, of course. We discussed how my body "buffered" me, and how I gave my power away to people. I realized that in situations like that, when I'm working with people who dominate the energy, I just want to disappear. Later I learned from a friend at work (the director) that the *woman who I was so threatened by had gone to great lengths to get me taken off the job. The director and I figured it was because she had been intimidated by me and my work.*

The story does have a good ending. Patricia gave me 2 days to meditate on thoughts of my body releasing weight and told me to thank it for protecting me. She also told me to let it know that I can take care of myself, that I no longer need it to buffer and hide me with excess weight! I was so excited when two days later, the weight was gone and I physically felt lighter!

I know I have the power to shapeshift now. I am practicing channeling the energy in a positive way. If I can move my energy in one direction, I can certainly move it in another. It just takes awareness and practice.

—Participant

Mental Laws

We often create conclusions about how the universe operates based primarily on what we understand, which often comes from our experience. When we have new experiences, we may in turn upgrade our conclusions. I find that the following four mental laws are valuable in teaching others to do what I did.

1. The Law of Consistency. In the FFF program, we will call what is consistently true for everyone truth. For example, if it were true that cookies make people fat, it would be true for everyone. Yet we can clearly identify many people who eat cookies whenever they want and do not gain weight.

2. The Law of Proportion. The more you think about something and experience the feelings, the more likely it is to manifest in your life or in your body. If you spend the day thinking negative thoughts about your body, and then say one positive affirmation that day, there's no question which reality has a better chance of manifesting. Rather than a food diet, try a mental diet.

3. The Law of Intensity. When you hold a thought with intensity, you get results that match your level of conviction. For example, some FFF clients who hear a new idea, such as "The body is mostly empty space" or "The body heals itself," have an "Aha!" experience that carries them successfully through the whole program. The "Aha!" creates a strong feeling that is connected to the new idea, and this stays with them over time. They hold onto that one thought and feeling with unwavering belief, and their bodies change as a result. This is what happened in the examples of shapeshifting in the previous section.

4. The Law of Like Produces Like. Thoughts are like seeds. In nature, when you plant an orange seed, you get an orange tree. Likewise, a lemon seed produces a lemon tree. It is impossible to plant an orange seed and get an apricot tree. This law of nature also exists within your mind. The seeds or thoughts you plant will be reflected in your physical form. Therefore, if you tell yourself "Everything I eat turns to fat" enough times, you will set that in motion. If you say "Everything I eat makes me thinner," you will create movement in a different direction.

In Conclusion

From the wonders of nature to the smallest subatomic particles that make up our bodies, we are surrounded by elements designed to respond to the thoughts we think and the pictures we hold. As you progress through the FFF program, you will discover new paradigms and skills that ask you to let go of destructive, self-defeating thoughts about food. You will enlist your mind to help you understand that food does not have the power to make you fat. Step by step, you will train your mind to create the reality you most desire so you can eat whatever you want and not gain weight. The possibility lies within.

PRACTICE SESSION 4

Visual Aid: On a piece of paper, write the following key words and place them as a visual reminder in front of you. For groups, place the paper in the center of the circle. For this chapter, the sign will say:

~ Your Thoughts and Beliefs Affect Your Body ~

1. Opening Attunement (see sample on p. 13 or p. 14)

If you so desire, light a candle to mark the opening of the session. I recommend that you play the subliminal *Freedom From Food* CD quietly in the background during the attunement.

2. Check-In (2–3 Minutes)

For Individuals: Write a page or more in your journal as a check-in with yourself. Next, review the topics that follow.

For Groups: Allow a 2–3-minute check-in per person. Tell a little bit about yourself and address the following topics. Speak about what has been working to change your thinking about food. (Remember to pass the talking piece and use a timer.)

• Share new insights about how the body heals itself (from Chapter 3).

• Share your answer to the homework question: What do you need to do to strengthen your connection to your Higher Self or Spirit to prepare for this FFF healing? What steps will you take?

3. 10-Minute Sharing

For Individuals: First read the following visualization. In your journal, write what comes up for you.

For Groups: This is a special time for one person (per session) to tell a personal story. It will allow you to get to know each person better. A lot of healing takes place by telling your story in the circle and having other people witness, support and deeply listen to you in a safe place. Remember, you need only share what you feel comfortable talking about. To begin, the leader can read the following visualization to the person whose turn it is. This will help you get in touch with what you would like to share.

Suggested Visualization to Assist the Sharing

I ask you to take a moment to close your eyes and connect with your heart. Now, I would like you to begin to follow the path that leads to your tears, pain, fear or any other emotion that connects you to your wound around food or weight (pause). Allow the important moments and events to come up (pause). Put an imaginary mirror up and look into it—not a physical look but an emotional one. What was your heart feeling then? What expression is on your face (pause)? Take a moment and let any other relevant scenes or feelings arise (pause). When you are ready, slowly open your eyes. If you are in a group, share your experience.

4. Appreciations

For Individuals: This is a good time to write down three appreciations of yourself— something about your essence. See the examples that follow.

For Groups: Three people from the group can give brief appreciations for the person who has just spoken. An appreciation should be something about one's essence—what you notice about that person. An appreciation should not give advice or include an explanation about how the person's story relates to your story. Here are examples of the kinds of appreciations you might offer:

I love your courage and the way you speak up for yourself.
I appreciate how you protect your Inner Child.
I think you are radiant, and I love your smile.

5. Break

6. Exercises

Go through the following topics one by one. Take 5–10 minutes to write your thoughts in your journal.

For Individuals: Review the answers you wrote.

For Groups: Go around the group to hear each person's thoughts. (Your timekeeper should allow each person 1–2 minutes to speak.) When everyone has had a chance to speak, go on to the next topic.

- Talk about messages you have received from other people that have had a lasting, positive or negative effect on you. For example, I mentioned how my mother was always telling me that I have a lucky star. Next, take a moment to go over what kind of thoughts dominate your thinking during the day. Are they judgmental, grateful, loving or depressed?

- Create an affirmation—a thought you want to consciously put into your mind to manifest the results you want. Affirmations are always in first person, and they are written in the present tense, as if they were happening now (for example, I can eat whatever I want, eat whenever I want and not gain weight. Everything I eat makes me thinner and thinner). Put these thoughts up around your house so they will be in front of you all the time.

For Groups: Allow a few moments to come up with an affirmation and then, one by one, share it with the group.

- Share what you are learning from your Inner Child work.

7. Practice Exercise—Reviewing Principles of the Mastery Keys

For Individuals: Journal your answers to the following topics. An understanding of the principles is essential to your 2-Week Healing process, so let the review really sink in.

For Groups: Go around the circle and speak about the following topics, one question at a time. An understanding of the principles is essential to your 2-Week Healing process. (Remember to pass the talking piece and use a timer.)

- In what ways is your body naturally self-healing? How does this help your weight issue?

- What have you seen in nature that supports the idea that you have a perfect proportion within you?

8. Homework

This week, your homework assignment is to do the following:

a. Write in Your Journal—What psychological work do you feel is needed for your healing at this time? Is it connected to self-esteem, setting boundaries, physical or sexual abuse, birth traumas, relationships, having children or some other issue? List any trauma that may be connected to your weight and log in what you plan to do about it in the next months (for example, get some kind of professional help).

b. Inner Child Exercise—Continue developing your relationship with your Inner Child daily by listening to the *Freedom From Food* CD (with audible words). Write in your journal what you discover.

c. Review the principles from the previous chapters and write a few sentences about each one.

- Diets Don't Work

- First Mastery Key—The Body Heals Itself

d. Mirror Work—This exercise can be done in 5–10 minutes. You begin by looking at yourself in the mirror and saying the things you have always wanted to hear about yourself and your body. These may or may not be things that you believe yet. However, your thoughts are powerful. Here are some examples I used when I was feeling ugly:

You are so pretty. You have the most beautiful hair and skin. People walk by and say how fabulous you look. You have the most magnificent eyes.

At the time I was saying these things to myself, I felt they were far from the truth. What I noticed, however, was that my outside world starting feeding back to me the thoughts I was creating inside. People would stop and say I was beautiful. At first, I thought that they just didn't see me and I was fooling them. Then I began realizing that I liked their vision of me far better than my own. I had a choice about which one to believe—I chose theirs. From that point on, I decided to always believe the most positive thought presented to me. Try it. You may be amazed at the results! The saying "Fake it till you make it" supported me while I went from negative thinking to seeing my positive beliefs manifest in the outside world.

e. (Optional) Skip ahead to the next practice session in Chapter 5 (for groups, choose one person to do this). Read Exercise 9 and, if you wish, prepare a tape in advance of the following session.

Reminder for groups: Choose a new leader for next week.

9. Appreciation

For Individuals: Write a few sentences in your journal about what most moved or inspired you in this chapter.

For Groups: Go around the circle. Speak about what most moved and inspired you in the meeting today.

10. Closing Attunement (see sample on p. 13 or p. 14)

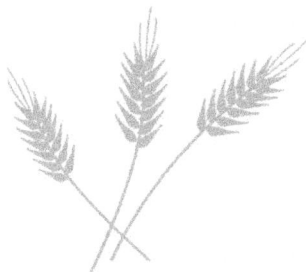

FIVE

THIRD MASTERY KEY:
EMOTIONS AFFECT YOUR BODY

I believe all emotions are healthy, because emotions are what unite the mind and body.... To repress these emotions and not let them flow freely is to set up a dis-integrity in the system, causing it to act at cross purposes rather than as a unified whole. The stress this creates, which takes the form of blockages and insufficient flow of peptide signals to maintain function at the cellular level, is what sets up the weakened conditions that can lead to disease.

—Candace B. Pert, PhD, *Molecules of Emotion*

The Wise Woman Speaks

You are now at the top of the mountain, ready to begin your descent into the shadow where deep emotions dwell. I want you to follow the inner trail that leads to your feelings and wounds of separation. It is time to look at situations and relationships that have caused you to split off from your essential self, your power and your heart.

It is these places that make you want to eat, hide and hold onto weight for protection. Your wounds create a veil, a cloud, a shroud of confusion from negativity and shame that covers the magnificence of who you really are. It is time for you to emerge and reclaim the special and unique gifts with which you were

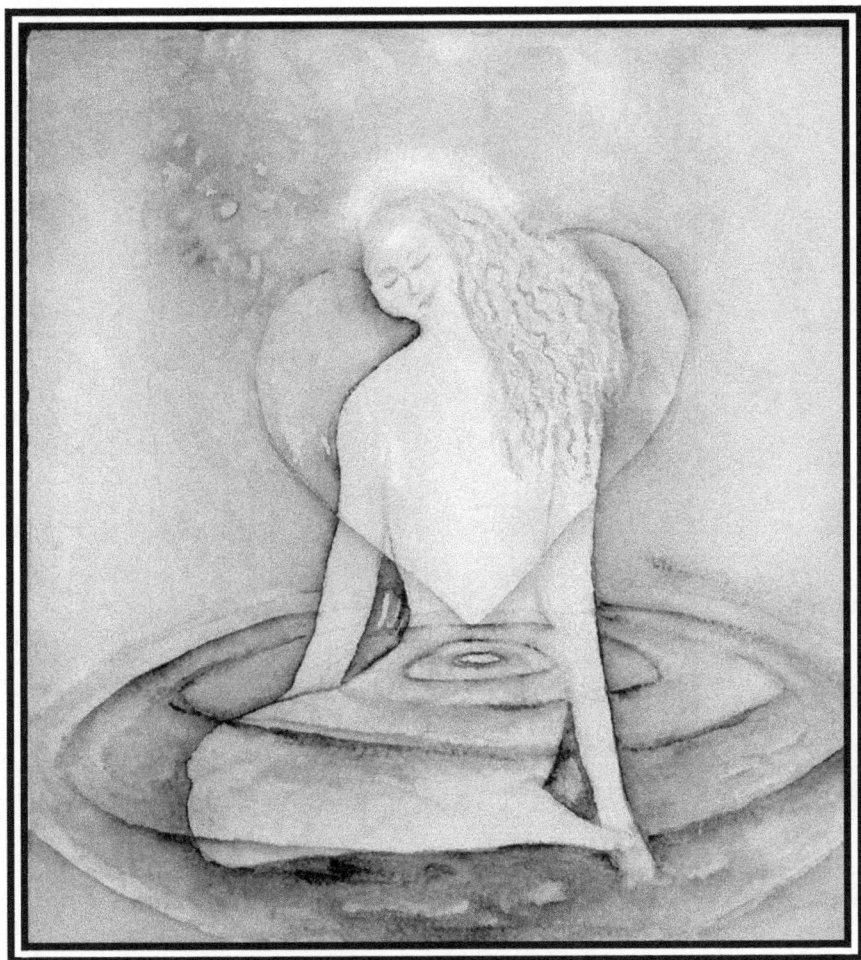

Reflections by Patricia Bisch

born. Remember, *emotions carry a powerful energy that causes fluctuations in your physical form. That is why you will be looking deeply into the **Third Mastery Key—Emotions Affect Your Body**.*

This part of your journey will light up the specific wounds you need to explore further. Then it will be up to you to do the psychological and spiritual work. The task is to find the way back to your open heart and into love once again. *For love is the emotional energy, the powerful universal force that unlocks the channels and flow in your body, releasing the blocks and contractions that cause weight.*

As you learn about this Mastery Key, you will have an inner knowing, a body sensation or some clear signal as to which emotional issues are still festering within you. It is always a journey into the dark, to feel and face your demons head on. "Will I come out alive?" you might ask. There are no guarantees. And yet to heal, you must go. It may involve enduring some anxiety, fear and grief. It is time to look into the shadow parts of yourself that dim your light.

Meeting the Shadow

The shadow is the part of yourself that lies beneath the neatly sorted appearance of your life. It is the dark lagoon of *emotional baggage* that has been following you around. There are many false layers built up so that to the average observer, you might seem to have it all together. Yet, in the deep caverns of your being, the wound still pulses, affecting your experiences and your choices. Degradation and devaluing yourself live and thrive here.

It is the discomfort of this core pain that causes people to search endlessly for an outside fix. Relationships, food, sex, work, alcohol and drugs are just a few of the things we use addictively to sedate our suffering. It is time to turn inward.

Connecting With Your Inner Child

People with food problems often feel emotionally *alone and unloved*. These are the feelings people eat over. This is usually caused from being disconnected from one's Inner Child, which affects the whole energy flow in the body. In *Healing Your Aloneness*, Margaret Paul and Erika Chopich speak about the Inner Child in relationship to the Inner Adult. These roles replicate the parent/child archetypal relationships that remain throughout life. Paul and Chopich write,

> *When these two parts are connected and working together, there is a sense of wholeness within. When these two parts are disconnected, however, because of being wounded, dysfunctional or undeveloped, there is a sense of conflict, emptiness and aloneness within.*

Geneen Roth, author of *When Food Is Love*, elaborates on the pain of the child.

> *We all have broken hearts. Every single one of us has had our heart broken at least once in our families, from the loss or betrayal of a parent. Some had their hearts broken over and over again in terrible ways. When the heart of a child is broken, something inexpressible and up to that moment whole and unquestioned snaps. And nothing is ever the same.*

Food is often a way we fill the emotional holes in our lives. We do it to survive and keep ourselves sane. It serves to sedate the devastating feelings of unbearable aloneness and abandonment. Food can be a replacement for parental love that was missing in childhood. Roth goes on to say,

> *Compulsion is despair on the emotional level. Compulsion is the feeling that there is no one home. We become compulsive to put someone home. Food was available when our parents weren't. Food won't abandon us, sexually abuse us, or criticize us.*

When children are not nurtured or cared for properly, they often feel they are not enough. It is not possible for them to acknowledge that anything is wrong with the adults on whom they are dependant. This would threaten their very existence. They must hold the adults as innocent. One way children do this is by persuading themselves that they are the reason for the problems.

Whether the challenges are related to their looks, intelligence, body or charisma, these children convince themselves that they are defective. They often go their whole lives as if under a spell, magnetizing different situations and relationships that substantiate their beliefs and self-judgments.

Are there any ways in which you can see self-judgment and inadequacy affecting your relationships or life situations? Take a moment now to go inside and contemplate where you don't feel good enough (pause). Until this wound of shame is healed, it will continue to be a formative undercurrent in your experiences.

Therefore, it is essential to learn how to listen to your Inner Child's needs and give her a voice. Simultaneously, it is important to develop the voice of your Inner Adult, who must learn how to nurture this Child. That is why I have recommended throughout the practice sessions to listen to the *FFF* CD segment about connecting with your Inner Child. Develop a relationship with her by having a dialogue every day. Pay attention to her complaints and find her underlying needs. See if they can be met and grieve together if they cannot.

Take the time to build a new bond with your Inner Child. By asking questions, you will begin to form a trusting rapport with her and find your way back to loving and valuing yourself.

Healing My Inner Child

Starting in my 30s, I began the journey of developing my own healthy Inner Adult. At first, I resented taking on a parenting job that should have been done by my father and mother. I felt that I had been an adult all of my life, taking care of my parents' disowned needs and protecting my sisters. I perceived that I had been robbed of my childhood, and now I was being asked to be a parent again, this time to myself. When would the time ever come for someone to take care of me and be interested in what I needed? However, there was no one else to do the job. My Inner Child was wounded and bleeding. I cared about her so I signed on, willing to build a personal relationship with her.

I remember journaling to get in touch with my Inner Child's feelings. In my first communication, she told me that she thought that I was very boring and that spending time with anyone else would be more exciting than spending time with me. She said that she felt completely alone in this life. Even when we were together, she felt disconnected from the whole world and experienced that no one knew or cared if she was dead or alive.

Weekends, mornings and late nights were her worst times. She was in constant pain and had little self-esteem, feeling not enough in any number of ways. Through lots of crying and desolate loneliness, I finally came up with some suggestions for how we might play together. The first one was to paint. I would take large canvases and just let her throw paint and express herself. My fingers and anything else around were fair game for our creative endeavor.

Don't get me wrong. This may sound like we were having great fun, but that would be very misleading. At first, it was just one step above pain—just OK and nothing more. However, I was willing to accept this baby step. We have continued to build our relationship in other projects, such as sculpting, painting and jewelry making, which even to this day are rewarding for us both.

Developing a bond with my Inner Child was not an overnight process. Her self-esteem was so low. I remember thinking for quite a long time that all the positive things I was doing were not building much of anything. It felt like there was a hole in the bottom of her boat.

At first, your Inner Child might react like a dog that has been beaten. When you put out your hand, she cowers. It can take awhile for an abused dog to trust that you are consistently going to be there for her and not hurt her. Therefore, when forming a relationship with your Inner Child, my advice is to stay with it and don't get discouraged. Every kind move you extend toward her does count and is making a difference, whether you see it or not. I patiently attended to her as long as she needed it, not expecting her to feel strong right away.

Everyone encounters situations that have not turned out the way they wanted. I grieved for the part of my Inner Child whose dreams got dampened. Now she often lets me know when things are not right, and I have learned to listen and respect her. I find great wisdom in her feelings and gut responses. Her emotional state is directly connected to my eating and to my body.

For example, I noticed over the years that when I broke up with a man, I went straight for candy and ice cream. It was my symbolic way of giving myself the love I was not getting. Feeling rejected and abandoned, I temporarily soothed the pain with something I could give myself.

Setting Boundaries

All children are dependent on the protection of the adults around them to survive. Drawing boundaries and creating safety are major emotional issues that face most overeaters. They generally do not feel they can say "No" when they need to. As children, they likely had to endure many forms of invasion into their personal space, emotionally or physically, which left them feeling defenseless and terrorized.

Objecting and saying "No" are natural for a child. Watch a healthy 2-year-old. One of the most primitive ways to get a sense of self is to be able to say, "I am different than you!" A healthy parent understands and values this process. Isn't it interesting that we live in a culture where this stage is known as the "terrible twos"?

Fearful of encountering shaming criticism or some form of violation, the Inner Child walks through life feeling vulnerable and open to outside attack. With ineffective parents to protect and nurture them, such Inner Children feel unable to object or draw healthy boundaries against the anger, judgments and rejections of others. The following are some examples of statements that create boundaries: "I don't like the way you are talking to me." "The tone of your voice scares me." "Stop speaking to me like you hate me." "Stop trying to run my life."

Anny Eastwood, MFT, who has been a specialist in eating disorders, explains that overly dominant, controlling caregivers are usually at the root of anorexia and bulimia. She says that when parents constantly insist, "I know what you think, feel and need better than you do," their children in essence have to learn how to swallow the caregivers' interpretations, even when they don't match the child's experience of herself. If verbal objection is not valued or welcomed, the objection is forced to go into "code"—a denser behavioral language that isn't as direct but means the same thing. Throwing up is one way to symbolically purge oneself of the toxic interpretations of others. Refusing to eat may be an attempt to take back control of one's own being.

Learning Assertiveness

Developing assertiveness is essential for people who are holding onto weight. Weight can serve as a boundary to keep people away. It becomes the unspoken words. In my classes, I do not applaud students for being nice guys at the expense of themselves. Instead, I give points for drawing good parameters. If you can protect your Inner Child by creating appropriate limits and saying "No" for her, then she will not need to use food to insulate and protect herself.

At first, you may think you sound harsh when you are speaking firmly and taking care of yourself. Firm is not mean. Setting boundaries and saying "No" when warranted are acts of true self-love.

As people with food problems, we are far too empathetic. We listen far too long and stay in uncomfortable situations much longer than is healthy so we do not hurt someone else's feelings. We think of this as being nice. This is not nice. This is being a doormat. It is so common for overeaters to be everyone's best friend. We will give you the shirt off our backs and do anything for you. We give and give to everyone except the one person who needs it most—ourselves.

You need to learn how to assert yourself and say sentences such as: "I need to go now. I am uncomfortable talking about this. I have only 2 minutes to talk now. I feel uncomfortable with the way you are talking to me. No, I need to stay home and take care of myself. No, No, No." Then your Inner Child will begin to feel safe and trust that you will take care of her. Try asserting yourself one time today and see how it feels. This is an important step to healing your emotions that connect to your weight.

Ask yourself how many times you defer to other people's needs and wants? Do you placate others and go along with things when you really don't want to? The truth is that if you do this, you will eventually resent it. And these resentments will come out in direct and indirect ways.

You may have to risk losing some people in your life. Superficial friends will fall away. Your real friends will stay around when you start to speak up for yourself. They will support and nourish your growth. True friends will also be happy for your successes and want you to be all that you can be. They will not want you to dim your light. They will see your success as confirmation that they can have more success, too. These are the kinds of people you want around you. It is your birthright to shine brightly. You do not have to give up yourself to be loved.

In the words of Marianne Williamson in *A Return to Love,*

Our deepest fear is not that we are inadequate.
Our deepest fear is that we are powerful beyond measure.
It is our light, not our darkness, that most frightens us.
We ask ourselves, "Who am I to be brilliant, gorgeous, talented, fabulous?"
Actually, who are you not to be? You are a child of God. Your playing small doesn't serve the world.
There's nothing enlightened about shrinking so that other people won't feel insecure around you.... We were born to make manifest the glory of God that is within us. It's not just in some of us...it's in everyone. And as we let our own light shine, we unconsciously give other people permission to do the same. As we are liberated from our own fears, our presence automatically liberates others....

People Pleasing and Caretaking

Some overeaters will try to do anything to keep the peace and not make waves, afraid to bear any more pain, anger or humiliation. They numb their feelings with food so they can appear OK. Without a biological or Inner Mother or Father creating safety, the Inner Child resorts to unhealthy tactics to keep herself safe.

One tactic is to become a people pleaser. This is a strategy of getting love and caring from another by foregoing and hiding your own needs. People who do this find the love they desperately need by adapting and becoming good little girls, being what their parents want. As children, they may get their parents' love by pleasing them. However, the adults really are loving the false self that these children have created, not the authentic child with her unique needs and individual characteristics. That is why she has such a sense of devastating loneliness.

Other children survive by acting out, rebelling, being chronically angry (always finding something wrong with someone else) or by being overly controlling. However, all of these behaviors in the end serve as survival coping mechanisms and need to be addressed.

Codependency

Many people with food problems suffer from codependency. This means being dependent on something outside of yourself for emotional well-being. For example, my self-esteem might rest on your opinions of me. If you love and approve of me, then I feel great. If you withdraw your love, don't like me or reject me, I feel that something is wrong with me. If you are not happy, I cannot be happy. Your needs are more important than mine, and I frequently postpone my own desires. Then resentment builds when I feel my needs never get met.

At gatherings, I often found myself overly concerned and occupied with other peoples' comfort to such a high degree that I forgot my own. I remember a great affirmation I used to help me break my codependent ways. It said, "I trust everyone to take care of themselves and ask for help if they need it." I started enjoying the social groups at my house much more. Try this affirmation and see if it makes a difference in your life.

Sexual and Emotional Abuse

Many eaters have experienced sexual abuse in the past. Extreme cases can terrorize a child to the core. When I began my psychotherapy practice, I was astonished to find out how many people were affected by such abuse. Having your boundaries violated can be like a soul robbery, after which you feel like your essential identity has been wounded. People often disconnect from their body emotionally and physically to survive and feel safe. This can interfere in your romantic and business relationships, ability to parent children, sexual life and so on. With a weak and undeveloped Adult Self, the sensuous, free, curious Inner Child feels defenseless against sexual or physical predators.

When you have been sexually abused, you get confused and can't think clearly. Often the abuser is a person who is someone you love or appears nice and friendly. This is what is so confusing. For survivors, it is often hard to tell friend from foe. Whom can you trust? Why did this happen? Who is to blame? Your instincts become wounded. It is difficult to know when someone is crossing your comfort line or your boundaries in general. Whereas a healthy person would know immediately that certain behaviors are unacceptable, in many instances you have trouble discerning what is appropriate.

There are various other reasons why people want to keep sexual advances away. Some camouflage their sexuality so they won't be tempted to be unfaithful to their partners. They know they do not have adequate boundaries. Some people gain weight as a response to being overly pressured to look good. These individuals are usually from families where physical beauty, popularity and being thin are the primary qualities of value. Who you are as a person doesn't matter. There are other scenarios where people were reprimanded for drawing any attention to themselves—showing beauty or sexuality was forbidden. Consequently, they never learned how to honor and beautify their body. There are so many ways the emotions around weight and sexuality are connected.

Take a moment now and ask yourself, "How is my body weight serving me? What is the message that it transmits to the world?"

To an emotionally abused child, the world also feels unsafe. Dysfunctional families create environments that can be filled with rage. Their homes are like war zones, where family members must walk carefully around topics that could contain hidden landmines. No one can be sure when or where the next explosion of anger may appear. Body fat is one way to insulate against hurt and pain. It can soften the blows. Food numbs the shaking inside and provides a way to survive repression and denial. It can dull the panic and be a distraction from the paralyzing shame that threatens to surface at any moment. This kind of relational environment is the breeding ground for lifelong hurt and deep resentments.

It is essential for you to find a way to explore these painful experiences—not just harbor them. Feelings are energy, and the nature of energy is to move and express. If you put a lid on emotional wounds, the pressure just builds and at some point there will be an explosion or implosion. This kind of denial always takes a toll on your body.

Expressing or connecting with suppressed feelings can seem dangerous and overwhelming to an overeater, however. It is difficult and crazy making when as a child you have been forbidden to speak about what is emotionally going on with you. Many children were given threatening statements if they dared to express any feelings at all, for example, "Stop crying or I'll give you something to cry about," or "If you keep this up, I'll take you to the orphanage."

The implosion that usually results from repressing emotions is extremely damaging. The sworn silence, like a spell, needs to be broken so that the memories and traumas can be healed. It can be a frightening process to uncover the wounds and be flooded by emotions that have been locked away for so long. This is why I want to mention again the importance of receiving professional help while you are healing your emotional scars.

Love Is Your Essential Emotional State

It is vital to find your way back to the resonance of love and an open heart, for these states are deeply connected to your body weight. Love is the essential ingredient of who you are. That's why you feel so seen and nourished when someone loves you or you cherish yourself. It is the real food.

As an infant, you come into the world with this pure resonance. It is noteworthy that your body usually exhibits its perfect proportion at this time. Emotionally, you are sensitive and open. That's why mothers are so protective of their newborns. It is important for mothers to be careful about how they hold their children and what tone of voice they use to speak to them. All outside sounds and noises send ripples throughout an infant's entire being. That's the sensitivity of the open, unguarded heart.

You can see more qualities of this pure, essential loving state by observing young children, kittens and puppies. Generally, they are not contracted, protective, shielded, shut down or disconnected. Inevitably, when I ask the people in my group to describe babies and toddlers, they say that they are trusting, cute, playful and so forth. A young child loves everybody. This is the state of being into which we are born and to which our inner current is always trying to return.

If depression and separation were a part of our natural state, we would be at home and happy in those feelings. Our inner voice would say, "Yes, I have finally arrived. I am sad all the time, anxious, fearful and separate from everyone." When we felt alone or in pain, we would know everything was right with the world.

Fortunately, this is not the place that feels most natural. When we feel depressed or disconnected from others, the driving force within instead pushes us to do anything we can to resume a state that feels happier and more connected. We meditate, pray, go to therapy, call a friend, walk out in nature, exercise, read positive books, write

—whatever it takes to restore our equilibrium. This is a similar force to the one that always pulls our bodies back to a state of health and our ideal weight, as discussed in Master Key One—the Body Heals Itself.

When I ask people to think of a time when they could eat whatever they wanted and not gain weight, it's no accident that they almost always think of a time when they were in love, carefree or creative and not even thinking about food. Take a moment and see if you can recall a time when you felt loved and seen and were not gaining weight (pause).

Why People Eat

The following list gives some reasons why people use food to sedate themselves.

1. To get affection, attention or love. (Food is something you can give to yourself to replace the love, touch or kind words that are missing.)

2. To numb anxious feelings. (Food can help you pretend nothing's wrong and protect your vulnerability.)

3. To shield or protect you from unwanted sexual advances, intimacy or abuse.

4. To deal with internalized anger, if you have no outlet or permission to be angry.

5. To feel some control in a world where things might seem very out of control.

6. To be obedient and avoid conflict.

7. To rebel against those who have tried to dominate you.

8. To reduce the pain of feelings of rejection and low self-esteem (not feeling good enough).

9. To help you feel better when nothing else is going right.

10. To camouflage fear and hurt from the outside world.

11. To compensate for childhood feelings of being left out and not chosen.

12. To alleviate boredom and loneliness.

13. To help with feelings of undesirability.

14. To deal with fears of success or failure.

15. To soothe feelings of helplessness and hopelessness.

In Conclusion

Negative trauma becomes crystallized in our bodies. To release weight, it is important to untangle the negative emotional webs that cloud our essential selves. We must keep patiently clearing emotional trauma until we regain our dignity, power and self-respect.

It is my experience that you do not have to heal all of your emotional problems to heal your weight issues. The truth is that healing your psychological self is a life-long journey. I was in my 20s and in therapy when I healed my weight, and I guarantee you, I had not resolved all my psychological-emotional issues. My self-esteem was still very low, and I had many layers of the onion left to peel.

How much a person has to work through varies. I tell participants to clear out just as much as they can in the period leading up to the 2-Week Healing. Although love and forgiveness are the goal, I recommend focusing on them only after you have found the root of the emotional decay in your life and cleaned it out. I hold the knowing that you too can find your way back to an open heart.

I am finally at a place in my life where I am able to open and have love even for the people who were my greatest tyrants. I feel safe in extending my caring, even if it is the smallest line of connection. It doesn't mean I have to be with these people or that I condone their behavior. I open my heart now because I understand that any part of it I close off prevents me from receiving the love I need.

PRACTICE SESSION 5

Note: It may take several weeks to complete the exercises in this session. Each week, repeat steps 1–4 and then continue where you left off with the exercises. Always close with the final appreciation and closing attunement.

Visual Aid: On a piece of paper, write the following key words and place them as a visual reminder in front of you. For groups, place the paper in the center of the circle. For this chapter, the sign will say:

~ Emotions Affect Your Body ~

1. Opening Attunement (see sample on p. 13 or p. 14)

If you so desire, light a candle to mark the opening of the session. I recommend that you play the subliminal *Freedom From Food* CD quietly in the background during the attunement.

2. Check-In (2–3 Minutes)

For Individuals: Write a page or more in your journal as a check-in with yourself. Next, review the topics that follow.

For Groups: Allow a 2–3-minute check-in for each person. Tell a little bit about yourself and address the following topics. Also, share how you are incorporating the new food principles into your life and what has been working to change your thinking about food. (Remember to pass the talking piece and use a timer.)

- Share your answers to the homework question: What psychological work is needed for your weight healing around self-esteem, setting boundaries, physical or sexual abuse, birth traumas, relationships, having children or other issues?

- Share the experiences you had while doing mirror work.

- Share any insights you've had about how your thoughts and beliefs affect your body (from Chapter 4).

3. 10-Minute Sharing

For Individuals: First read the following visualization and then write in your journal what comes up for you.

For Groups: This is a special time for one person (per session) to tell a personal story. It will allow you to get to know each person better. A lot of healing takes place by telling your story in the circle and having other people witness, support and deeply listen to you in a safe place. Remember, you need only share what you feel comfortable talking about. To begin, the leader can read the following visualization to the person whose turn it is. This will help you get in touch with what you would like to share.

Suggested Visualization to Assist the Sharing

I ask you to take a moment and close your eyes and connect with your heart. Now, begin following the path that leads to your tears, pain, fear or any other emotion that connects to your wound around food or weight (pause). Allow the important moments and events to come up (pause). Put an imaginary mirror up and look into it—not a physical look but an emotional one. What was your heart feeling then? What expression is on your face (pause)? Take a moment and let any other relevant scenes or feelings arise (pause). When you are ready, slowly open your eyes. If you are in a group, share your experience.

4. Appreciations

For Individuals: This is a good time to write down three appreciations of yourself—something about your essence. See the examples that follow.

For Groups: Three people from the group can give brief appreciations for the person who has just spoken. An appreciation should be something about one's essence—what you notice about that person. An appreciation should not give advice or include an explanation about how the person's story relates to your story. Here are examples of the kinds of appreciations you might offer:

I love your courage and the way you speak up for yourself.

I appreciate how you protect your Inner Child.
I think you are radiant, and I love your smile.

5. Break

6. Discussions

For Individuals: In your journal, write answers to the following topics.

For Groups: Go around the circle and talk about the following topics. (Remember to pass the talking piece and use a timer.)

- Discuss the main points in this chapter that are of interest to you.

- Share what boundaries you need to set in your life. (Remember, it is not self-loving to take care of others' needs and not get your own needs met.)

- Share about the Inner Child work you are doing.

- Discuss where you see yourself as codependent and one thing you could do differently to change.

- If you feel comfortable and it applies, you can share how sexual or emotional abuse has affected your weight.

7. How to Handle the Emotion of Anger (Exercise on Assertive, Passive and Aggressive Behavior)

a. Begin by reading the following descriptions:

- *Assertive behavior* is a healthy way to handle your anger by stating your wants and needs, while respecting another person's wants and needs. It is possible to speak honestly, but not hurtfully. By asserting yourself, you will build your confidence and self-esteem. You will teach others how to treat your feelings in a respectful way. Of course, it is important to discern the appropriate circumstance in which to assert yourself. If you are too assertive with your boss on a job, for instance, you could be fired or perceived as a problem. However, in most situations, asserting yourself will be the most self-loving and effective form of communication to get the most desirable response available.

To begin asserting yourself, start your sentences with *I statements*. For example, you might say, "I felt uncomfortable when you were late. I feel frightened or put down when you talk to me that way. I felt accused when you looked at me that way." Stay away from *you statements* that tend to point the finger at the other person. Examples of such statements are "You made me angry," "You are the reason I'm sad," or "It's your fault that I got fired." It is also important to tell the other person what you would like. Examples are "I felt hurt when you said that to me, and what I would like is for you to apologize." "I am angry that you are late again, and I would appreciate it if you would call me when you are not going to be on time." While assertive behavior is honest and direct, it is never disrespectful.

• *Aggressive behavior* is harsher. It occurs when you state your feelings directly in a way that violates the rights of other people or intimidates them. It does not have regard for another's feelings. Aggressive behavior sometimes gets results, at least at the moment. However, it almost always incurs retaliations or feelings of revenge. Expressing anger in this way creates a false sense of power and control. Those who constantly run over others and ignore their feelings lose in the long run because people do not want to be around them. For example, when a clerk in a store charges you the wrong amount, an aggressive response would be to call the person names and say something such as, "You are so stupid! You idiot! Don't you know how to do your job?"

• *Passive behavior*, on the other hand, seeks to avoid an immediate conflict. Often people are passive because they do not want to experience anger, disapproval or abandonment from another person. Passivity involves agreeing to do things you don't want to do. Saying "Yes" when you mean "No," saying you will do something you have no intention of doing or not saying anything are all passive moves. Although you may avoid conflict, passive behavior fuels resentment and in the end causes more ill feelings than telling the truth. So learn how to get the courage to speak up for yourself.

In conclusion, assertiveness is more effective in producing healthy results than the other two options. However, that doesn't mean assertive behavior will always help you avoid unpleasant feedback from people. Still, your responsibility is to let people know how you are feeling and what you are thinking in the healthiest and most respectful way. You are not responsible for their reactions. Being willing to speak the truth takes courage when you feel that you are at risk of losing love. Every time you speak truthfully, you will gain a deeper sense of personal power, which will eventually allow you to handle situations more effectively. The best gift from your new actions is that your Inner Child will feel safer, and she will trust that you will draw boundaries for her. This can reduce her need to hold onto weight for protection.

b. Now, write in your journal the three situations where it is most difficult for you to say "No." Are you generally assertive, passive or aggressive?

c. Next, make up assertive statements you could say in those situations.

For Individuals: Write your answers in your journal.

For Groups: Come back into the group. Share your answers and check if the whole group agrees that your answers are assertive.

d. Next is a practice session to demonstrate your new skill.

For Individuals: Practice imagining there is a person asking you for a favor and your assignment is to say "No" to her no matter how she tries to manipulate you. Next, make up assertive statements for similar situations and practice saying them aloud.

For Groups: Pair off and practice asking each other for a favor. The person who is being asked needs to practice saying "No" to the request, no matter how the other person tries to manipulate her. Share in the group what comes up.

8. How to Handle Emotions That Occur From Being a Rescuer, Victim or Persecutor

Karpman Triangle Exercise

(To begin, read the following pages that explain the Karpman Triangle):

In psychology, the Karpman Triangle is frequently used to show how we switch among the roles of victim, rescuer and persecutor and the emotional components of each position. I present it here because many overeaters who grew up in troubled families get trapped in this pattern. Unfortunately, it often gets played out later in relationships until it is recognized and resolved. This triangle is somewhat like a board game. There are three players—the victim, the rescuer and the persecutor. The goal is to get healthy. You can do this by finding your way out of the triangle.

The *victim* is the person on the board who acts out feeling hopeless, helpless and needy and who appears not to be able to function well in this world.

The *rescuer* takes on the victim's responsibilities, feeling sorry for her. The rescuer believes that the victim truly is incapable of doing things for herself. Therefore, the rescuer may defend her, make excuses for her, do things for her, cover for her, do her chores and give, give, give to her emotionally.

The *persecutor* is the person who feels angry. She may yell or resentfully pull back and withdraw from the relationship. She ends up feeling used, not taken care of, unfairly blamed for her caring and help. She often feels ostracized and may feel guilty. Her needs are not met and she feels very frustrated by this.

You may find yourself starting in your life in any of the positions in the triangle. For this section, I have mostly taken the position of the rescuer to explain how the game works. The game and pattern start when someone on the board starts rescuing a person. They begin seeing the other player as incapable of taking care of herself. The rescuer starts doing things for the victim, such as covering for her, overhelping, taking on confrontations that need to be made and so on. Both people begin colluding in the helplessness scenario. At first, the victim sings the rescuer's praises. She might imply that you are the only one who can save her. However, the turn in the game is soon to come.

At a certain point, the victim starts getting angry and starts blaming you (becoming the persecutor). She wants you and your good intentions to stop interfering with her life. She resents being seen as someone who cannot take care of herself and resents you for butting in with your so-called help, telling her what to do. She may ostracize you and become angry. You, the rescuer, now feel victimized, unfairly accused, not taken care of or appreciated (you become the victim). This dance continues round and round the triangle. Does this sound familiar?

The endless cycle stops when the rescuer stops rescuing and allows the other person (acting as victim) to be responsible for her own life, feelings, predicaments and actions. As children, we were dependent on our parents. As adults, we are generally capable and responsible for taking care of ourselves. So when people need help, rather then rescuing them, offer the phone number of a good professional and allow them to take (or not take) the necessary steps.

You can throw out a life jacket to someone drowning, but you cannot make the person put it on. You can lead a horse to water, but you cannot make it drink. We cannot know what is best for someone else. We can offer assistance, and then we must let go and trust that each individual is making the perfect choices to learn what lessons are needed. We cannot play God. By holding in your consciousness that as adults we have the ability and the responsibility to help ourselves, we honor each other and release and free ourselves. We stop enabling the part of another that is a victim and start affirming a person's capabilities. This is the winning move on the board, the way out of the game.

Quite often people will be angry when you pull yourself out of the game and stop rescuing. They have depended on you to play this role. You may be ostracized or have to endure their blame or anger for a while. I do not want to give you the impression that this task is always easy or without ramifications. However, it may be the price you have to pay to free yourself and reclaim your life. I recommend that you create a lot of support and love to help you through this transition.

Next, answer the following questions:

• Do you see yourself as a victim, rescuer or persecutor in a triangle?

• If so, what steps do you need to take to get out and get healthy?

• Write in your journal (or share in your group) what you see as your predominate pattern in the triangle.

9. Sexuality Exercise (This is an exploration of the emotions connected to your sexuality.)

For Individuals: Read the following visualization aloud or (play the tape if you have made one). Play some music in the background as you listen to the tape. Have your journal and a pen ready to write down your insights and experience at the end of the exercise.

For Groups: Choose one person to read the visualization aloud (or play the tape if someone has made one). Put on some music in the background, softly enough that you can still hear the person reading. After the exercise, take time to silently write down your insights and experience and share them with the group.

Visualization

…Stand up and close your eyes. Just for a moment, imagine you are free from all limitations, roles you play to hide yourself and the shoulds and should nots others have tried to impose on you (pause). As you begin to feel this, let your body begin to move in a way that expresses this freedom. Feel the free child part of you begin to move in an uninhibited way, joyfully connected to the innocence of who you really are. Let the part of you that's bursting to be alive come out. Allow your body to move sensually, if that arises (pause).

As you physically express yourself, be aware of any movement that you feel you must inhibit. Observe any embarrassment connected with it. In front of whom would you find it most difficult to do this movement? As you continue, see that person in front of you now. See in what way the person is judging you (or you are judging yourself) that makes you want to contract (pause). Feel the pain and shame you have lived with that restricts you from moving freely and expressing yourself. Watch how you stop the flow of your body so that you might get acceptance, love or approval.

Next, tell this person, silently to yourself as you continue moving, that you are no longer willing to restrict yourself. Allow yourself to begin to move more freely, even if in a small way and with less holding back. See how good it feels not to stop yourself anymore (pause).

(If you are working individually, visualize different people in your life as you walk around in the next part.) Now, walk around the room and do not shut down. Connect with people while you move. If you again have the desire to turn yourself off, remind yourself that you've now taken your power back. You have the right to move freely and feel good in your body. If others are uncomfortable with it, that is their problem. You will no longer close yourself down for them. Know that you also have the right to move sensually in any way that feels good to you (pause).

Now, you can very slowly begin to come to a stop. Allow yourself to review the things that you want to remember from this exercise. In silence, get a pen and journal and write about what came up for you in this process. If you are in a group, you can take some time to share your experiences.

10. Homework

This week, your homework is to do the following:

a. Inner Child Exercise—Continue developing your relationship with your Inner Child daily by listening to the *Freedom From Food* CD (with audible words). Write down in your journal what you discover.

b. Review the Mastery Keys and principles from past chapters. Write a few sentences about each one of the following:

- Diets Don't Work

- First Mastery Key—The Body Heals Itself

- Second Mastery Key—Mind Creates Matter

c. Practice drawing boundaries and asserting yourself. This will create safety and send the message to your body that it no longer needs protection from extra weight. Say "No" when it is appropriate. You receive extra credit for any time you are not just being a nice guy or allowing others to walk over your own feelings and needs. Remember, being firm is self-loving, and assertive is not aggressive. For now, it is better to err on the side of being overly strong in your statements than to negate your needs.

d. Bring different kinds of food to the next meeting. Include things such as candy and cookies as well as foods such as carrots and fruit.

Reminder for groups: Choose a new leader for next week.

11. Appreciation

For Individuals: Write a few sentences in your journal about what most moved or inspired you in this chapter.

For Groups: Go around the circle. Say what most moved and inspired you in the meeting today.

12. Closing Attunement (see sample on p. 13 or p. 14)

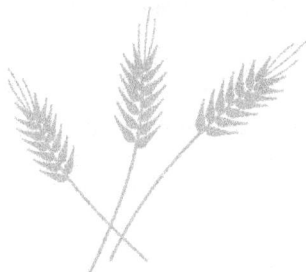

SIX

FOURTH MASTERY KEY: FOOD IS ENERGY

As Einstein taught us, mass and energy are differentiated principally by form. Your body is a form of energy slowed down to assume the appearance of mass. And the mind directs the energy that determines the form. You do have the power to create the form you desire to live in. Don't forget that your body, as well as everything physical in life, is an effect of a prior cause. The cause is in your mind where you direct the energy flow. The beliefs and attitudes you hold about yourself and your life are manifest in your body.

—Terri Cole Whittaker, *What You Think of Me Is None of My Business*

The Wise Woman Speaks

You are now ready to take the next step of this journey. Take my hand as we go deeper into the forest. Let yourself begin to resonate with the natural surroundings. We will rest at this clearing where a circle of stones surrounds a very old tree. I want you to focus on the ancient tree standing directly in front of you. There are words written on the trunk, but they are invisible to the naked eye.

I invite you to close your eyes and allow me to lightly touch them. This will enhance your vision instantly, creating a new lens through which to see. Next, open your eyes. You now have the ability to decipher the words on the tree, *Fourth Mastery Key—Food Is Energy*. Allow your consciousness to expand as you begin to contemplate and drop into the vast reality of this idea.

~

Food and Air

To help you further grasp the concept that food is energy, think of food as if it were air. Air is light and permeable and has no apparent substance. You ingest it continuously in great quantities, and it just passes in and out of you unobstructed. *Food is a mindless, nonintentional, neutral energy.* You would never think air would cause you to gain weight. You simply take it in and release it while breathing, without attaching any other thoughts to it.

This is how small children relate to food, unless they have been programmed otherwise. They often eat all kinds of sugar, candy and cookies, never thinking they will gain weight—and they don't. They don't even know what a diet is. It is no accident that people who are thin take in and release food in the same way. They never think food will make them fat. They always tell you that no matter what they eat, they never gain weight and they don't know where it goes.

Therefore, release your consciousness from thoughts that are binding. Let food begin to flow in and out of you unobstructed, like the air you breathe. It is your thinking and beliefs that cause food (light energy) to stabilize as weight. Without interference, what you eat can decompose very quickly. Become aware of what you are cultivating and growing in the garden of your mind. When you are eating, begin to play with the concept of this Fourth Mastery Key. Although you are not ready just yet to go out and eat anything you want, you can begin changing your consciousness right now.

Everything Is Energy

As we view the nonmaterial world, we are exploring *everything as energy*. We are examining our essence, the pure consciousness that exists before form as well as our ability to create from this nonactualized place. Our body, cells and the food we eat are composed from this unified, living energy field that is continuously changing. It is from here that our ideas create and coagulate into what appears as matter.

Whether it is chocolate cake, an apple, a chair or a rock, it is all energy directed by your mind. Energy cannot think or have bad intentions. A chocolate cake cannot decide to make one person gain weight and another person be thin. In and of itself, a cake cannot make you do or be anything. It certainly has no brain. This is the conceptual reality on which FFF is based. (If you are saying to yourself, "Yes, but what about calories and metabolism?" that will be addressed in a few pages.)

Similarly, sugar has been given a bad rap. We are taught that it has the power to make us fat. If that were absolutely true, then I believe all people would get heavier from it. However, many people eat sugar and stay thin. They may not feel great, which is another issue, but they don't necessarily gain weight.

A brownie has no more power over you than a carrot stick. In this paradigm, they are both mindless energy that would go right through you and be eliminated—if you did not interfere in the process with your beliefs. From the perspective of the Freedom From Food program, the ideas and emotions you hold around the brownie cause it to affect your weight. Your thoughts have the power to make the brownie's influence negative or positive, healthy or unhealthy.

Your Body Is Energy

Your physical form, as well as everything you see, is really just energy slowed down or speeded up, which differentiates how it appears. Remember Deepak Chopra's statement: "You change your body more effortlessly, more spontaneously and more expeditiously than you can change your clothes." He said that you are literally changing the atoms that become cells of your body every time you breathe in and out.

Therefore, begin to let go of the old thought that your weight will never come off. Replace this view with how changeable your body really is. This will open you to the possibility that you do have the control and ability to rearrange your figure by carefully choosing your beliefs. Just as one small breath can disperse a whole dandelion and one small pebble can send ripples throughout a pond, a single thought can create fluctuations in your body. Try visualizing the atoms that compose your physical form as bubbles of energy that move easily. Picture weight leaving your body like champagne bubbles leaving a glass.

Years ago, I saw Kirlian photography that captured on film the concept that we are in fact energy beings. The photographs showed that we have an energy field around our body, called an aura, which is not perceptible to the naked eye. Our auras change all the time. It is an illusion that our bodies stop and are finite, solid, material form. Scientists have discovered we are mostly empty space as well. Take a moment and feel the difference when you perceive your physical form as mostly empty space rather than dense matter.

The Power of Your Thoughts

Often people will say, "I'm not eating more food. I'm hardly eating anything at all, and I'm still gaining weight." This is true for them, but it is really not food that is making them fat. In *The Incredible Cosmic Consciousness Diet*, Harvey Cohen, PhD, pointed out that when we believe in perfect health, the *energy* of that thought will cause our body to react to make it so. He said, "Your mind will always find a way to create the realities of your beliefs...." According to Cohen, this explains why:

- Some people remain healthy no matter what kinds of food they eat.

- Some people remain slim no matter how much "fattening" food they eat.

- Some people remain overweight no matter how many diets they go on.

In the material world, where most peoples' consciousness resides, food and weight become sluggish and stuck. People feel victimized and entrapped by the food they eat. They are unaware of the power of their words. They don't understand that the real trap is in what they are thinking. Their thoughts are what command the energy that must comply. When people say, "Oh, this ice cream will go right to my hips," they are sculpting the energy right in. Then they blame the ice cream! We believe we can joke with our friends and call ourselves ugly and fat and say mean things to ourselves without consequences. However, the subtleties of our words are registering on us and in us all the time.

If it were life or death, we wouldn't fool around this way. What if someone said, "If you tell yourself even one more time that food will make you fat, you will get cancer." You would stop, wouldn't you? You would see the seriousness of what you were saying and the life-or-death effect of even casual comments. You would not give yourself the permission to flounder recklessly with your thoughts. You would realize the cost—your life.

With food, however, we think we can get away with it. We slap our thighs and instill our thoughts, solidifying the energy. We say, "Look at these fat thighs; look at this fat stomach," and we feel our rolls. This horrific self-judging becomes embedded in our physical form. We rampage our body temples and defile the jewels. We tear down the sacred. Our statements have much more power than we give them credit, and the ramifications are vast. It is time to be much more mindful of our thinking and what it creates.

The Epiphany

When I really understood from taking Nick's class that food and my body are just energy, it was an epiphany for me. It catalyzed a huge shift in my consciousness and opened unlimited possibilities. This "Aha" experience was an awakening in my healing journey that would change my understanding of food and my body permanently.

Different foods no longer had the power to make me gain

weight. I did not evaluate them as "good" and "bad." I started perceiving my physical form and food as porous, spacious, weightless and mutable. All excess food would blow off me and through me effortlessly, like a subtle breeze.

Years ago, I heard about a man named Jack Schwartz, a yogi who could put a knitting needle repeatedly through his arm. The puncture wounds closed immediately and were completely healed in 24–48 hours. This was fascinating to me. I concluded that to do this feat, Jack must have mastered the concept that his body was not solid, but a mass of energy slowed down. His accomplishment substantiated for me the new insights about food and weight that I was discovering.

Rethinking Calories

I am often asked, "If food is energy, what about calories?" Thirty years ago, when I was first developing the FFF program, I decided to look up *calories* in the dictionary. Webster defined *calories* as "heat units of energy." That was astounding to me. It did not say fat units or weight units of energy.

I thought about how this would apply to foods with a high caloric count, such as pecans or candy. According to the definition, when people eat high caloric foods, they are taking in more heat energy than they would get from other foods. Since we are not hibernating, we do not need to store heat. Therefore, I deduced that our body would eliminate excess calories automatically. This was a completely new way of conceptualizing for me that was aligned with my new understanding. By the way, I also discovered that carbohydrates are organic compounds of energy and that fat is stored energy.

Try it out. Picture yourself eating something that is filled with calories and guaranteed to make you gain weight. However, this time picture yourself eating the same food but visualizing it as heat units of energy. See yourself ingesting it and your body naturally releasing the excess heat energy. Notice how different this feels.

Rethinking Metabolism

What about metabolism? We are taught that if you have a high metabolism, you burn up calories quickly and that if you have a slow metabolism, you store the calories as fat. Doctors say the rate of metabolism is regulated by our physicality and exercise. However, Nick taught me that from his experience and understanding, metabolism is regulated by the mind. My own healing and work with people over the years substantiates this.

I have observed that when people hold completely to the FFF principles for the 2-Week Healing, they make a quick shift in how they process the food they eat. They ingest significantly more calories, exercise less or not at all and do not gain weight. Their body seems to be burning off higher amounts of calories, and the only thing that has changed is their thinking. I regard this as evidence of a body/mind connection and proof that consciousness can change metabolism.

In Conclusion

From this point forward, you need to visualize food as neutral energy, whether it is junk food or health food, pizza or apples. It is time to let go of old perceptions about which foods will make you gain weight. Start seeing all food as energy, light and empty space instead of dense matter and enjoy how different you feel when you eat!!!

PRACTICE SESSION 6

Visual Aid: On a piece of paper, write the following key words and place them as a visual reminder in front of you. For groups, place the paper in the center of the circle. For this chapter, the sign will say:

~ Food Is Energy ~

1. Opening Attunement (see sample on p. 13 or p. 14)

If you so desire, light a candle to mark the opening of the session. I recommend that you play the subliminal *Freedom From Food* CD quietly in the background during the attunement.

2. Check-In (2–3 Minutes)

For Individuals: Write a page or more in your journal as a check-in with yourself. Next, review the topics from Chapter 5 that follow.

For Groups: Allow a 2–3-minute check-in, where you address the following topics taken from Chapter 5. Also, share what has been working for you this week to change your thinking about food. (Remember to pass the talking piece and use a timer.)

- Share times you were assertive and drew boundaries this week.
- Share any new insights about your sexuality and food.
- Share any new insights about the Karpman Triangle.

3. 10-Minute Sharing

For Individuals: First, read the following visualization and then write in your journal what comes up for you.

For Groups: This is a special time for one person (per session) to tell a personal story. It will allow you to get to know each person better. A lot of healing takes place by telling your story into the circle and having other people witness, support and deeply listen to you in a safe place. Remember, you need only share what you feel comfortable talking about. To begin, the leader will read the following visualization to the person whose turn it is. This will help you get in touch with what you would like to share.

118

Suggested Visualization to Assist the Sharing

I ask you to take a moment and close your eyes and connect with your heart. Now, I would like you to begin to follow the path that leads to your tears, pain, fear, shame, anxiety or any other emotion that connects you to your wound around food or weight (pause). Allow the important moments and events to come up (pause). Put an imaginary mirror up and look into it—not a physical look but an emotional one. What was your heart feeling then? What were you needing? What expression is on your face? What is your posture like? Tune into how you are breathing (pause). Take a moment and let any other relevant scenes or feelings arise (pause). When you are ready, slowly open your eyes. If you are in a group, share your experience.

4. Appreciations

For Individuals: This is a good time to write down three appreciations of yourself—something about your essence. See the following examples.

For Groups: Three people from the group can give brief appreciations for the person who has just spoken. An appreciation should be something about one's essence—what you notice about that person. An appreciation should not give advice or include an explanation about how the person's story relates to your story. Here are examples of the kinds of appreciations you might offer:

I love your courage and the way you speak up for yourself.

I appreciate how you protect your Inner Child.

I think you are radiant, and I love the way your eyes light up the room.

5. Break

6. Discussions

For Individuals: Write in your journal about the topics that follow.

For Groups: Go around the circle and speak about the topics that follow. (Remember to pass the talking piece and use a timer.)

- Share the points in this chapter that you found to be most important.

- Share what you now understand about food being energy.

- What directs the food energy that you eat? How does it work?

- What are calories? How is metabolism connected with weight?

7. Practice Exercise

This is a deepening exercise to help you know that food is really mindless energy and cannot make you do anything. Food has no intention because it doesn't think.

First, make little stations around the room where you put different foods, such as chocolate chips, apples, nuts and crackers. Also, place in the stations some inanimate objects, such as rocks, a chair and a pencil. Remember to include the practice of eating air. Since air is energy, too, most people never think that it will make them gain weight no matter how much they eat.

For Individuals: You will speak aloud both parts of the exercise. First, ask yourself the questions for the exercise and then answer them.

For Groups: The leader will ask the following questions as she holds up different inanimate objects or food from the various stations. The whole group will reply.

a. Demonstration One for the Exercise (If you are in a group, this will be done together.)

The leader will hold up something that is considered health food, such as a carrot. Ask the group, "What is this?" Members of the group should answer, "Energy." (Prompt them if necessary.) Then you can ask, "Does it have a mind? Can it make you do anything?" Then hold up some type of junk food, such as candy, and after that, an inanimate object. Ask the same questions. You should get the same kinds of answers. The leader should repeat that it is all nonintentional, mindless energy without a brain.

b. Demonstration Two for the Exercise

Pick two people to demonstrate the exercise to the whole group. (If you are doing this as an individual, you will play both parts.) Call them Partner A and Partner B.

Partner A asks one question at a time:

"What is this?" (hold up a pencil, then a cookie)

"Does it have the power to make you do anything?"

"Can it make you stand up?"

"Does it have a mind?"

"Does it think?"

"Does it have intention?"

"Can it make you gain weight and make another person not gain weight?"

"Does it have a brain?"

Partner B answers with the Mastery Keys and principles from the program. She will respond with information, such as

"That pencil [or cookie] is mindless, neutral, nonintentional energy and has no ability to command me to do anything. If everything is energy, then it does not make sense to label one item as bad [weight producing], while something else, such as a carrot, is labeled good [slimming]. It is our mind that makes it good or bad."

c. The Exercise

For Individuals: Speak aloud both parts of the exercise. First, ask the following questions and then answer them.

For Groups: This exercise is done in pairs. Pick a partner and choose who will be A and B. In the example that follows, Partner A is called Pat and Partner B, Susan.

Partner A Pat says, "Chair, make me gain weight."

Partner A continues, "Susan this chair can't make me gain weight. This chair can't make me do anything because _____." (She substantiates this by explaining something she has learned from the chapter. For example, her reason could be that a chair has no mind or ability to intend, and therefore, it can't make her do anything.)

Partner B Susan acknowledges her, saying, "You're right, Pat. This chair can't make you gain weight because _____." (State another reason you have learned, for example, that the chair is just energy without a brain.)

Continue going around to the different stations until you have completed them. Then switch roles (Partner A becomes Partner B) and repeat the exercise. Next, return to the circle and share your experience. Although it may seem a little silly, people inevitably report that they have profound changes from doing this exercise.

8. Homework

This week, your homework assignment is to do the following:

a. Listen to the first track of the *FFF* CD (the opening visualization) and see if you can really understand that food is energy. Whenever you are eating, begin to see food as mostly space and not solid, dense mass. See it as "light," like bubbles in a champagne glass. Visualize what you eat as being airy, easily moving and changing shape, like the seeds of a dandelion that disperse with just a small breath.

b. Inner Child Exercise—Continue developing your relationship with your Inner Child daily by listening to the *Freedom From Food* CD. Write in your journal what you discover.

c. Review the principles from past chapters and write a few sentences about each one.

- Diets Don't Work
- First Mastery Key—The Body Heals Itself
- Second Mastery Key—Mind Creates Matter
- Third Mastery Key—Emotions Affect Your Body

d. Have a magazine day and cut out different pictures that reflect the body you would like to have. Superimpose your face on the image. This will give your body the road map of the state to which it is returning. Visualization sends your body the message to begin to rearrange itself, which can affect your metabolism. Remember that energy flows where your attention goes; therefore, put your attention on images of your slim body.

e. Draw a picture of yourself thinking negative thoughts, feeling attacked from the outside or feeling closed in and contracted in your body. Show how the food energy gets stuck when you are imploding in this way. Then draw another picture of yourself feeling open and safe with your energy flowing. This picture should depict food (energy) going in and out of your body unobstructed. Use these images as visual reminders when you need to change your thinking.

Reminder for groups: Choose a new leader for next week.

9. Appreciation

For Individuals: Write a few sentences in your journal about what most moved or inspired you in this chapter.

For Groups: Go around the circle. Speak about what most moved and inspired you in the meeting today.

10. Closing Attunement (see sample on p. 13 or p. 14)

PART III

EMPOWERMENT TRAINING

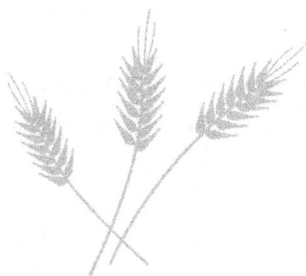

SEVEN

SABOTEURS

*Great spirits have always encountered violent
opposition from mediocre minds.*

—Albert Einstein

*If you open yourself on one side, or in one part, to the Truth, and on
another side, you are constantly opening the gates to hostile forces, it is
vain to expect that the divine Grace will abide with you. You must
keep the temple clean if you wish to install there the living Presence.*

—Sri Aurobindo, *The Mother*

The Wise Woman Speaks

There is a serious expression on the Wise Woman's face. She
looks into your eyes in a way you have never seen before. With sober
urgency in her voice, the Wise Woman speaks:

I am proud that you have made it through the Four Mastery Keys
and follow-up practices. You have unlocked the understanding to
begin the next step. The 2-week test of fire is coming up, and it
will call on you to give 100 percent of yourself.

You must be ready on all levels, so we will begin preparing for this
empowerment. It is necessary to wake up and learn how to show
up for yourself. To assist you in this process, I call on the following

Goddess Archetypes and strong Animal Symbols known to destroy that which is out of alignment with what is believed to be true: Dragon, the High Priestess, the Warrioress, the Protector, the Tiger, the Jaguar, Kali and Pele. You are going to have a meeting with yourself and the outside world that will be transformational. However, attempting to do the 2-Week Healing without proper preparation would be like skiing down an advanced slope or skydiving without adequate training.

Listen carefully to what I have to say. You are in danger. Your Saboteur is killing you off, and you don't even know it. It is stalking you, waiting for the perfect moment to steal your power and bring back doubt, self-loathing and shame. This part of you wants to take your strength and tell you that you are nothing. It wants to sabotage your efforts and say you will never have what you want in life, no matter how hard you try. You will always be overweight, and nothing is ever going to change. *Meet your Saboteur.*

The Battle of Good Versus Evil

Ever since Eve was tempted in the Garden of Eden and ate the apple, we have been subject to sabotaging thoughts of good and evil. We have the free will to choose, and free will is a tremendous responsibility.

Saboteurs have been identified and recorded in many forms throughout history. We have heard fairy tales such as Little Red Riding Hood, where the Wolf is dressed in grandmother's clothes and is ready to eat the little girl, and modern stories such as Star Wars, where the evil power of Darth Vader challenges the light of Obi-Won Kenobi.

We all have within us sabotaging thoughts of destruction, separation and competition that fight against healing thoughts of peace, love, oneness and union. In a world filled with new technology, good ideas can easily be corrupted by nearsightedness, greed and power. The best of intentions can be undermined when they are not thought out carefully.

For example, the atomic bomb, an innovative idea to keep our country safe, has produced toxic waste that could kill us in seconds. Because of our shortsightedness, the world is contaminated with massive amounts of nuclear fallout that will silently threaten our lives for the next million years. With new technologies such as cloning coming to the fore, we need to see the bigger picture and develop more scrupulous ways of tending the ideas we create.

One of the greatest obstacles to the success of the FFF program is the inability to be vigilant about the ideas by which we live. Our thoughts about our body are not exempt from the imperative need for discernment. We must closely examine all ideas we hold about food and weight, for every one will influence our body's health and perfect proportion. *Whatever we focus on will expand.* Our thoughts can be cataclysmic or plodding, healing or transformative—whatever they are, they will affect us.

What Are Sabotaging Thoughts?

In this program, sabotaging thoughts are detrimental, unloving beliefs about yourself and your body. They feed on your shame, self-judgment and hopelessness. These thoughts are slimy. They want to block any change that might make your life better. New ways of being just don't feel safe to these parts of you. They are the bowels of your thinking. Their comfort lies in outmoded survival strategies that worked in the past. Their goal is to have you give up your dreams, agree that you are just too damaged and die.

Destructive thoughts may come from your internal voice or an external voice via family, friends, the media and so forth. To succeed in your 2-Week Healing, it is essential to learn how to deal successfully with them. You must start looking and deeply listening with mindfulness to your inner conversations. Mindfulness is an ancient Buddhist practice of staying in the moment with thoughts, feelings and actions. In this program, we will be using a type of vigilance to stay awake to our sabotaging thoughts.

To begin, *take a close look at any place in your life where you feel that energy might be leaking or drained by your internal dialogue.* The following are some examples of Saboteur voices that you can recognize and intercept when you sharpen your attunement.

Critical Saboteur

This negative, critical voice always wants to remind you that you are not enough. It sounds something like this:

You are undeserving. Everyone else will get this program but you. You should give up hope. You are not smart enough, pretty enough, thin enough, intelligent enough, charismatic enough, compelling enough, successful enough. You are just plain not enough!!! You are defective.

The Critical Saboteur reminds you that any part of you that feels good or gets what you want is just a temporary imposter that sooner or later will be exposed. The truth will be revealed that you really don't have what it takes to be loved, accepted or successful. It will stop you just before the finish line. You will be found out, and all the good things you are trying to hold onto will be taken away.

Scientific or Lawyer Saboteur

This voice keeps finding scientific and intellectual evidence for why the FFF program doesn't work. It finds opposing thoughts by authorities that tell you this program is faulty. You will know this is a Saboteur because, when given a sound reason why its thinking doesn't hold up, the next doubting thought will soon come forth. The endless stream of these ideas signals this as a negative pattern for you.

If this is happening, you won't be able to stand solidly behind your new belief system. Instead, your inner voice will be running the show. The opposing evidence it presents will sound convincing until you learn and practice in this chapter and in the next one how to listen carefully. For example, it will say things, such as

"I just heard about a study saying that carbohydrates definitely

cause fat," or *"I just read an article that says exercising three times a day is the only way to get thin."*

This voice will constantly find another way to keep you thinking that what you are learning is wrong. Therefore, you will never have a chance to stand behind any positive new ideas long enough to see if they work.

Impatient Saboteur

This voice will say things such as,

This program is taking way too long, and besides I just found a quick and easy weight loss plan on the Internet. We need to be thin by the wedding or the summer or some other event. We can't fit into our clothes; we have nothing to wear. We can't wait forever for this program to work! We need results now!

The Impatient Saboteur shows you where you are not perfect in your body and points out that you are overweight. You end up feeling that you cannot take another minute of this condition. Instead of sticking with the program, you start to feel that you better go on a diet and lose weight now—even though you've been down that road countless times in the past and it hasn't worked. Everything this voice has to say sounds like a child's tantrum. The message is *"I want what I want now, and anything else just isn't good enough!"*

"Yeah But" Saboteur

"Yeah but"s are the food of this insatiable Saboteur. They are like the question "Why?" to a child. *Why is the sky blue? Why is the earth round? Why is the sun yellow?* The "why, why, why" becomes endless. Although it is positive to answer these imposters up to a point, eventually, too many questions produce a negative effect. The "yeah but" voice will make it impossible for you to ever come to a conclusion, make a commitment or hold a proactive stand. *It is the never-ending nature of the questioning that lets you know this is a Saboteur.*

Naming Your Saboteur

In the practice session at the end of this chapter, you will be asked to write a page or two naming your Saboteur. This will enable you to become fully aware of this part so its dialogues of doom no longer fool you. The following is an example of a sabotaging voice from a past participant in the FFF program:

———

Bitter Betty

I am that voice in your head that keeps you feeling not good enough. You are not to have what others have…because you don't deserve it. Those opportunities are available to "other" people; they are not intended for you. Look around…you are a pair of brown shoes and the rest of the world is a tuxedo.

The reason you feel uncomfortable in social situations is because you know you aren't interesting to talk to. You don't have anything to offer and no one really cares what you have to say. And you never seem to have the right thing to wear. Since you don't have a nice body…if you dressed a little "hipper" or more stylishly…that would certainly help…but you just aren't attractive to men. You don't dress feminine; you are frumpy, overweight and you have no sexual energy… Men feel comfortable around you because you pose no threat. Sure, you can make them laugh and you are a good listener, but that's about it. You will always be just a "friend" to them…nothing sexual…you are just not appealing.

Your clients like you for the same reason. Having you around makes them feel prettier, thinner and more attractive…. You are safe and don't pull the focus from them, and they like that.

Face it…what you want doesn't really matter! You've gotten way more in this life than anyone else in your family…so just be happy! Marriage isn't for everyone… So what if you don't have a relationship or children of your own…you have a career and you've traveled. Try appreciating what you have in life rather than thinking about what you want. You want far more than you deserve anyway. Who do you think you are? Most people don't even notice you, and if they've met you…they don't even remember! The sooner you just accept you will always be fat, single and alone…you will be able to live the life you are supposed to have and stop all that silly dreaming.

—Participant

Instinct Wounding

Most overeaters in this society are *instinct wounded*, which leaves an open door for Saboteurs to enter. They don't notice when their own thoughts or someone else's thoughts are negatively affecting them. Picture a mouse or a bird oblivious to the danger of a nearby cat. *An unaware bird will not sense that the cat is preying on it.*

In our society, women seem to be more instinct wounded than men. Because they are raised to be empathetic and nurturing, even if their own needs have to be put on hold, they are afraid to lose love if they draw healthy boundaries. For example, they won't stop a friend from talking about diet plans and calories. Instead, trying to be nice, they let in sabotaging ideas that food will make them fat. This throws them off course in the program. As an overweight eater, you need to develop a stronger awareness about how you allow in unhealthy messages.

The following are examples of how instinct wounding may show up while you are in this program:

• A television show is talking about diets (Saboteur to this program). You are unaware of the messages going into your consciousness, and you don't change the channel.

• You focus on how women look after they lose 50 pounds quickly on a diet and conveniently forget how often they gain the weight back and more. Your impatience gets fed and you again start entertaining a quick fix, forgetting your lifetime of failures in dieting and keeping off the weight.

• A friend starts talking to you about a diet, and you don't notice that the information is creating doubt about this program, which you are currently trying to complete.

• You unconsciously listen to someone say that the ice cream you are eating is going straight to your hips, forgetting the direct effect thoughts have on your body.

• You read a magazine article on the latest diet, unaware that its messages are informing your cells.

• You go back to that situation where your food problems began and are once again surprised when you feel worthless, unloved and invisible. You begin feeling overlooked and not valued when your needs aren't being met. You return shattered and bewildered. Quickly you reach for food to sedate the pain and nurture yourself so that you can begin to rebuild your self-esteem. You conveniently plan your visit right at the time you are doing your 2-Week Healing. This disrupts your hard-won attempts to be strong and show up for yourself.

• You trick yourself into thinking you must do a fast, telling yourself you are just doing a cleanse when you are really dieting to lose weight.

...All the while your Saboteur is smiling, hiding in the corner...

The Threshold of Change

Major breeding grounds for Saboteurs are the places in your life where real change is possible. Why do they hang out here? Saboteurs are determined to keep you from making a breakthrough. Often in this program, they will wreak havoc on your new ways of thinking and tell you this process is a bunch of baloney—especially when you are about to do the 2-Week Healing and even after you have successfully completed it. If they do get your attention, you will find yourself consistently reeled back into loops of outmoded negative thoughts that lock up your energy.

Why does this happen? One of the main reasons is that, unconsciously, it might feel safer and more comfortable to play small and stay in the same pattern, where you don't get clobbered for shining. As children, we are taught that dimming our light can be a way to survive abusive situations.

Although most people say that they drastically want to change and will do anything to free themselves from their horrible addiction, when it really comes down to it, they find numerous reasons not to show up for themselves and this program, succumbing to these voices of doubt. It is not easy to change a pattern that has been with you for a lifetime. That is why you must learn how to ward off your Saboteurs.

Healthy Instincts

When you are healed, a solid front protects you from internal and external sabotaging voices. You have impenetrable boundaries to voices that would rob your new focus. You refuse to let unhealthy thoughts come in. You are not polite or bargaining about it. For example,

- You change the television channels that are counterproductive to this program.

- You are not afraid to walk out of the room if dieting or unhealthy conversations are going on.

- You remember the hell you once lived in and that it is only thoughts away.

- You realize that you do have a choice to open or close the door to different ideas, to accept or reject them. You have no intention of listening to or entertaining sabotaging thoughts.

- You carefully choose to be in relationships that make you feel seen and valued and that support the positive changes you are trying to make.

When your instincts are sharp and healthy, you have the ability to be alert. You can see this trait in wild animals. They are highly sensitive. The cat and the bird are aware when either one is near the outskirts of its boundaries. They have an innate, peripheral vision that senses danger closing in. As another example, think of what a deer does when a human or threatening animal approaches. The deer stops and listens astutely. There is a pregnant silence, full of signals about what is coming. It is almost as if the deer's breathing has stopped and its adrenaline is rushing. The deer is alive and fully present in the moment.

This is the type of alertness you will be developing. I am like this when anyone even begins trying to convince me that food will make me gain weight. I block anything that conflicts with my inner knowing and invades my consciousness with doubt. I am not open to any Saboteurs. In the next chapter, you will learn many tools to assist you in holding this kind of focus.

Tap Your Saboteurs Away

Tapping is one of the self-help tools professionals use to handle sabotaging, negative voices. This is a great way to banish "yeah but"s, mind chatter and blocks caused by conflicted feelings. For example, you try to lose weight, make more money or have a love relationship, yet *unconscious, underlying thoughts may counteract getting what you want.* Although you may feel you do all the right things, something still seems to block you from achieving what you desire. That is, you may consciously want to lose weight, but deep inside, you might unconsciously feel you don't deserve it. You may want weight to come off but also feel you need it for protection. As the well-known physicist Chilton Pearce said in the *Biology of Transcendence*, we need "unconflicted behavior" to achieve changes in our lives.

Tools such as tapping will assist you in staying aligned in your thinking so you can produce the outcomes you desire. Tapping acupuncture points can help alter the energy configurations that are held together by negative beliefs. Tapping releases blocks and opens up new pathways, allowing you to manifest new thought. If you are interested in exploring more of this work, you can look up Emotional Freedom Techniques (EFT) and find a practitioner in your area.

Gloria Arenson, MS, MFT, in *Five Simple Steps to Emotional Healing*, wrote about tapping the "Karate Chop Spot" to break up old emotional patterns. She described this spot as the fleshy part on the outside of your hand below the little finger (see illustration below). In the Freedom From Food sessions, participants have found that tapping just this one point helps to quiet their minds when they are feeling flooded with negative voices about food. Although there are more extensive applications to tapping, I will explain how to use just this one simple tool.

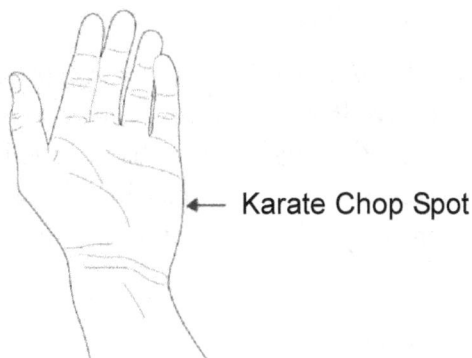

← Karate Chop Spot

First, as Gloria suggests, you will identify the negative emotion you are feeling. Second, you will add the phrase that you deeply and completely accept yourself. Third, as I personally recommend, you will add a positive phrase.

Repeat the entire statement (as shown in the following example) three times with as much feeling as you can, while you continually tap the Karate Chop Spot. Try to tap out your negative feelings in this way whenever you need it. You will always use the same phrases to begin your statements. They are as follows:

1. *Even though* I have this problem (*put in your problem*) _____,

2. *I deeply and completely accept myself* (just add this phrase),

3. *and I know* (add a positive phrase)_____.

Here are some examples of what to say while you are tapping your Karate Chop Spot:

- *Even though* I am afraid that everyone else will get this FFF course but me, *I deeply and completely accept myself…, and I know* that I am getting exactly what I need to succeed in this program.

- *Even though* I think to myself that this course is a hoax, *I deeply and completely accept myself…, and I know* that it is not a hoax because there have been times in my life when I have eaten whatever I wanted and not gained weight before I ever came to this class.

- *Even though* I feel that it is not safe to be thin and that I can't protect myself or draw boundaries, *I deeply and completely accept myself…, and I know* that I have been drawing boundaries more since I have been in this program and that I am building the perfect protection that my Inner Child needs.

In Conclusion

One way to recognize a Saboteur is to ask questions about the thoughts that are presenting themselves. Is there any productivity in exploring the question your mind is bringing up? Have you already answered that question many times? Is this thought just creating needless doubt or undermining your ability to succeed?

Stay aware! It is time now for vigilance and mindfulness in your thinking. You must develop healthy instincts to discern whether your thoughts and beliefs are beneficial or sabotaging. Don't give your Saboteurs a chance! Keep your awareness sharp and use tools such as tapping to keep them at bay.

PRACTICE SESSION 7

Visual Aid: On a piece of paper, write the following key words and place them as a visual reminder in front of you. For groups, place the paper in the center of the circle. For this chapter, the sign will say:

~ Vigilance, Mindfulness, Awareness ~

1. Opening Attunement (see sample on p. 13 or p. 14)

If you so desire, light a candle to mark the opening of the session. I recommend that you play the subliminal *Freedom From Food* CD quietly in the background during the attunement.

2. Check-In (2–3 Minutes)

For Individuals: Write a page or more in your journal as a check-in with yourself. Next, review the topics that follow.

For Groups: Allow a 2–3-minute check-in, where you tell a little bit about yourself and speak on the following topics. If something else is more pressing in your life, please also share that. (Remember to pass the talking piece and use a timer.)

• Share the pictures you created from the magazines that reflect you in the perfect proportion to which you are returning (homework from Chapter 6).

• Share the pictures you drew that show your energy both contracted and flowing.

• Share your insights about the Mastery Key that Food Is Energy (from Chapter 6). Do you notice any change in how you are relating to food? (Keep this new consciousness alive in you!)

3. 10-Minute Sharing

For Individuals: First read the following visualization and then write in your journal what comes up for you.

For Groups: This is a special time for one person (per session) to tell a personal story. It will allow you to get to know each person better. A lot of healing takes place by telling your story into the circle and having other people witness, support and deeply listen to you in a safe place. Remember, you need only share what you feel comfortable talking about. To begin, the leader can read the following visualization to the person whose turn it is. This will help you get in touch with what you would like to share.

Suggested Visualization to Assist the Sharing

I ask you to take a moment and close your eyes and connect with your heart. Now, I would like you to begin to follow the path that leads to your tears, pain, fear or any other emotion that connects you to your wound around food or weight (pause). Allow the important moments and events to come up (pause). Put an imaginary mirror up and look into it—not a physical look but an emotional one. What was your heart feeling then? What expression is on your face (pause)? Take a moment and let any other relevant scenes or feelings arise (pause). When you are ready, slowly open your eyes. If you are in a group, share your experience.

4. Appreciations

For Individuals: This is a good time to write down three appreciations of yourself—something about your essence. See the examples that follow.

For Groups: Three people from the group can give brief appreciations for the person who has just spoken. An appreciation should be something about one's essence—what you notice about that person. An appreciation should not give advice or include an explanation about how the person's story relates to your story. Here are examples of the kinds of appreciations you might offer:

I love your courage and the way you speak up for yourself.
I appreciate how you protect your Inner Child.
I think you are radiant, and I love your smile

5. Questions

For Individuals: Go through the questions that follow one by one. Take 5–10 minutes to write your answers in your journal.

For Groups: Take 5–10 minutes to journal your answers to the following questions. Then go around the group to hear each person's thoughts. Your timekeeper should allow each person 1–2 minutes to speak. When everyone has had a chance to share, go to the next topic. Go through the questions one by one.

- What are the sneakiest sabotaging thoughts you have had? Remember, they come disguised to appear as though they are helping you.

- How are your Internal Saboteurs critical of you? This program? Anything else you try in your life?

- Do your Internal Saboteurs find other material or other viewpoints to keep you from ever feeling firmly committed to this process (Scientific Saboteur)? Do they introduce nutritionists, scientists, doctors or other professionals with opposing viewpoints?

- Do your Internal Saboteurs flood your mind with unending "yeah but" comments?

6. Break

7. Tapping Exercise

For Individuals: Work on your sabotaging thoughts by saying them aloud, one at a time, while you tap your Karate Chop Spot. Follow the format in the examples that follow.

For Groups: Go around the circle and take turns working on your sabotaging thoughts. Practice tapping your Karate Chop Spot as you speak. Do three group rounds. For example,

- Even though I am afraid that everyone else will get this FFF course but me, I deeply and completely accept myself...and I know that I am getting it no matter what this negative voice is saying.

- Even though I feel that it is not safe to be thin and that I can't protect myself or draw boundaries, I deeply and completely accept myself...and I know that I have been drawing boundaries more since I have been in this program. I am getting better and better all the time.

8. Homework

This week, your homework assignment is to do the following:

a. Write 1–2 pages describing your Internal Saboteur. Give your Saboteur a name (review the example in the section on Naming Your Saboteur, this chapter).

b. Inner Child Exercise—Continue developing a relationship with your Inner Child. Every day, tune into your Inner Child by listening to the *FFF* CD section on this topic. In your journal, write what you discover.

c. Rent the movie *A Beautiful Mind* and prepare to discuss how the main character holds a focus and fights off his Inner Saboteurs. *Drop Dead Fred* is also good, if you can find it.

d. Review the principles from the past chapters. Write a few sentences about each one.

- Diets Don't Work
- First Mastery Key—The Body Heals Itself
- Second Mastery Key—Mind Creates Matter
- Third Mastery Key—Emotions Affect Your Body
- Fourth Mastery Key—Food Is Energy

e. Bring food that is high in calories or scary for you to eat to the next practice session.

Reminder for groups: Choose a new leader for next week.

9. Appreciation

For Individuals: Write a few sentences in your journal about what most moved or inspired you in this chapter.

For Groups: Go around the circle. Speak about what most moved and inspired you in the meeting today.

10. Closing Attunement (see sample on p. 13 or p. 14)

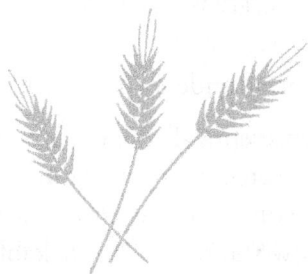

EIGHT

TAKING A STAND

*Until one is committed, there is hesitancy, the chance to draw back,
always ineffectiveness. Concerning all acts of initiative (and creation),
there is one elementary truth the ignorance of which kills countless
ideas and splendid plans. The moment one definitely commits oneself,
then providence moves too. Multitudes of things occur to help that
which otherwise could never occur. A stream of events issues from the
decision, raising in one's favor all manner of unforeseen accidents,
meetings and material assistance, which no man could have dreamt
would have come their way....*

—W. H. Murray, *The Scottish Himalayan Expedition*

*Whatever you can do or dream you can, begin it.
Boldness has genius, power and magic in it.*

—Goethe

The Wise Woman Speaks

Continuing on your journey, you accompany the Wise Woman
to a small clearing in the forest. She draws a circle on the ground and
within the circle draws a square. The Wise Woman begins to speak:

—

This circle represents the unified field of consciousness you will
be holding during your 2-Week Healing. It is the container for

143

the full, rich spectrum of understanding you have been learning.

The square inside represents all the corners of your body/mind, which will be totally protected in every direction from sabotaging thoughts. This new consciousness provides the proper "ecosystem" in which to grow the strong, unshakable, sustainable roots that are required to change your physical form permanently.

In this next passage of time you are going to learn how to *take a stand*. To do this you will discover how to hold and maintain a line of nondual thinking long enough to alter the subatomic particles of your body. When that happens, your body can change the way it processes food, so you no longer gain weight from eating. You do have the power to generate and sculpt the mass of light energy that is your physical form. The commitment necessary to hold a powerful stand has to do with three elements— your sense of knowing, sense of focus and sense of trust.

~

A Sense of Knowing

Most likely there are situations in which you already take a stand. In these situations, you hold in your mind a sense of knowing without doubt that life will always respond with an outcome that is congruent with your thoughts. For example,

- Do you always know you won't get sick in the midst of contagious influenza?

- Do you know a parking place will always be there when and where you want it?

- Do you have an inner clock you set with your mind and your body always wakes up at the preset time?

Take a moment and think of situations in which you already take a stand or have a knowing about something. These are situations where you have solid beliefs and certainty that you can consistently manifest things you desire.

For example, when people say, "I always get a parking place if I want it," they have no doubt about it. They seem assured that they can accomplish what they intend. They do not question themselves. You will see them create the desired conditions over and over again. These same people may be filled with doubt and insecurities in other areas of life, but in this one arena they are completely confident. What are some situations you encounter where you have a strong and solid stand about what you intend?

Holding a Focus

The film *A Beautiful Mind* is a powerful illustration of how someone can hold a focus to fight off those inner sabotaging voices. The lead character, played by Russell Crowe, is mentally ill and takes on the goal of returning to normal life. In a final scene, his negative, destructive voices manifest as several people whom he has created in his delusional mind. Appearing real, they stand on either side of him (as Saboteurs), wanting him to engage in conversations that seem relatively innocent and helpful. Their appeals are meant to engage him at his weak, emotionally vulnerable points. They are luring him back to his confused mental state so he will return to his illusionary way of thinking. What they are saying used to be compelling and important. Now he knows they have nothing at all healthy for him to hear. He understands that any response to their statements will be an open door for their sabotaging voices to come in and take over.

Therefore, he holds his focus on the path he is walking. Although he hears and sees the people, he manages the tension and *blocks out* their voices. He closes off to the feelings they are trying to evoke in him, which would pull him into destructive conversations and fog his brain. He *keeps his focus and his thoughts on the path*. (In our process, this means staying aligned and connected with the Four Mastery Keys.) In this state of intense presence, self-defeating thoughts cannot take hold.

Finally, he succeeds in evolving to a new place in his life. He is free from the anguish as long as he does not release his stand and go back to his old way of thinking. This is a taste of how it will be when you have to walk through the land of sabotaging thoughts during the 2-Week Healing.

Eckhart Tolle, author of *The Power of Now*, gives another example of holding a presence in the moment. He likens this state to walking a tightrope, where it is essential to be fully aware of what is happening at every step. All that exists is "this step." In the moment of now, all negative self-talk and the problems it attracts disappear. They fall away, unable to survive the environment of intense presence.

Finally, in speaking about focus, I want to mention neurolinguistic programming (NLP), which was founded by John Grinder and Richard Bandler in 1975. It is a study of the patterns created by the brain (neuro), language (linguistics) and the body. In neurolinguistics, eye movements in certain directions are studied to ascertain how they connect to one's thinking.

Eye focus can be of great assistance for holding a stand and fighting off Saboteurs. The following is an exercise that can help you understand the importance of the connections among eye focus, emotions and your body.

Exercise: First think of something sad…and give yourself time to feel this in your body. When you are feeling it, freeze the direction your eyes are looking (pause). Are they staring up or down? Take a moment and make a mental note as to what you were feeling and where your eyes were focused.

According to NLP, when people are feeling sad, they usually look down. It is not a surprise that people will say at times, "I feel down today" or "I feel depressed." The area around the stomach is the emotional center of the body, where feelings and self-doubting voices enter. Your body, in this case your eyes are following your thoughts. (I have observed that in some cases the eyes may look straight ahead when doing this exercise. However, I have never seen them go up.)

Now, take a minute and don't think of anything at all. Stop and check which direction your eyes are staring…up or down? According to NLP, when people are told not to think of a feeling at all, their physiology will generally follow by looking up. Perhaps that's why people use the phrase "Cheer up" to change someone's mood toward lighter, happier thoughts. Or they may say, "I'm feeling up today," meaning they feel good. (Once again, I have observed that in some cases the eyes may look straight ahead when doing this exercise.)

Therefore, when you are holding your stand and not wanting sabotaging thoughts to enter, focus up or straight ahead. Until now, you have been doing the beneficial work of digging up and clearing out old emotional traumas connected to gaining weight. However, during the 2-Week Healing, it is imperative that you do *not* explore those feelings, which can provide an entrance for Saboteurs.

Building Trust and Faith

During the 2-Week Healing, you will build trust in the Mastery Key principles. You have gained understanding of them, but now you will have to risk, *taking a stand* and testing them on yourself. For example, it is necessary to trust that your body will eliminate all excess food and not turn it into weight while you eat things that have been pronounced forbidden. It is the time of the unseen mystery of creation, where the formless (as thoughts) creates a change in the form (your body). No matter how much you know intellectually, you will need to jump into the unknown. It can be scary. Faith is a strong component of what will carry you through.

Your situation might be likened to that of a caterpillar, who does not know she will be transforming. The *imaginal cells* (which hold the image of her ideal form) are inside her but are dormant. During the time of cocooning, she is totally unaware that her body is changing. In fact, she appears to be dying. Then unexpectedly, she turns into a butterfly. It seems to be somewhat of a mystery or a miracle, but actually a natural process is going on all the time. (For more about this process, see *Butterflies* by Norie Huddle, which was published on Earth Day, 1990.)

In the 2-week FFF program, you start by mindfully putting into your consciousness new thoughts and principles (which are like the imaginal cells of the caterpillar). This occurs at a constant rate until a transformation begins in your physical form. Similar to the caterpillar, you may have no idea what is happening behind the scenes. You may wonder if the program is working or if your body is actually eliminating the food you are taking in. Often participants in this program ask, "When does the shift occur that I will no longer gain weight from food?" The answer is, you will not know. The shift happens in a moment *when you are not looking*.

Therefore, stepping on the scale or checking how your clothes fit is a big taboo. These backward steps of doubt inevitably stop the whole metamorphic process, and you may need to start all over again. The following are some ways people interrupt the process by checking:

1. Some people check by looking in the mirror.

2. Some people check by putting on old clothes that fit them when they were thinner.

3. Some people check by feeling into their body and registering if they feel like they have gained weight.

4. Some people check by getting on the scale.

To hold a stand, you must control your impulses and refuse to act on doubt or fear. Instead, replace such thoughts with trust and faith. Then in 2 weeks, when you get back on the scale, you will realize your body has changed and you are no longer gaining weight from food. You may have even lost weight. You have transformed into the butterfly.

Finding Your Warrioress

You have a strong, fierce and empowered part of yourself that is a Warrioress. She fights for your life and draws boundaries. She protects your heart and what you believe in and value. This is the part of you that shows up over and over again for your Inner Child, no matter what.

You need to get in touch with your Warrioress, for she is the one who is going to hold an impenetrable stand, taking you through the

2-Week Healing. In the practice session following this chapter, you will be asked to identify and write about her. Here are some examples written by former participants:

Catherine the Great

She is the part of me you better not cross unless you are ready to surrender. She will always win. She leads and unites. She leads me into and through fears that unite all my parts, the strong and the weak. She protects me from corrupt energy. She created boundaries for me and is consistently aware of my needs. She conquers all negative thoughts, even the faint whispers. She beheads all Saboteurs; no evil will disrupt our path. She is the perfect balance of strength and grace. She is virility and sensitivity in absolute harmony. She is sexual and powerful. She is committed to our journey of enlightenment. We seek love, truth, clarity and fulfillment through Divine guidance. She is my Warrioress. She will let me accept nothing but victory—a victory that will give me freedom. Freedom From Food.

Shananzia

My Warrioress essence is a powerful shaman who protects me at all times. She is strong, agile and fluid in her body. She can shapeshift easily and become invisible at will. She can move with the elements, calling the wind, summoning the rain, conjuring fire and opening the earth. She can set a circle of stones and call forth invisible allies to her side. Her weapon is her voice. Through sound she can stop her enemies in their tracks. She can create a ring of sound that is impenetrable. She can throw her voice to sound as if it is coming in a different direction. She can make the sounds of the fiercest animals to instill fear. Through her knowledge and love of the natural world, she can become any animal. Through her sensitivity, she can sense danger and disappear before it comes near. She

*can soar like an eagle or walk silently like a mountain lion. Her
name is Shananzia.*

Using a Coach to Prepare for Your Stand

We all have male and female characteristics within. The female
side is more intuitive, receptive and allowing. She sees what wants to
emerge. The male side of us moves forward and puts ideas into
motion. It is the part that protects us and our creations. That is why
we are now going to call on the male, Warrior/Warrioress part of you.

In general, men find it easier to take a stand than women. They
are groomed to be warriors, who are protective and mark boundaries
around their territory. At some time in their life, most men train
with a fierce coach in some sport or activity. They learn to pay attention and stay focused and alert. Part of their training is to thoroughly study every strategy and sneaky move of their opponent. They are
carefully taught how to dissect and counter every play. Millions of
dollars are put into their professional games, which they take very
seriously.

Think of the Lakers basketball team. The players understand that
during a game is not the time to be emotional but instead ready and
prepared. They have practiced their moves with great discipline and
are primed to defend their goals by keeping impenetrable boundaries. Doing whatever it takes to succeed, team members are totally
present to what is happening in every moment. They are not listening to outside comments such as, "Oh you'll never make that shot."
Cheers of yea and nay become background noise. The players understand that other people's thoughts and opinions are distractions that
will take them off their mark. It will be essential for you to access this
kind of astute awareness during the 2-Week Healing.

That is why, from here on out, I will take on the role of a coach
who reinforces the fundamental skills needed to complete the healing process. However, I can stand with you only if you are willing to

show up for yourself. I am calling on the *woman of power* who lives inside of you. It is necessary for you to step out of the part of your personality that doesn't feel good enough and finds reasons to play small. As your coach, I want you to be totally consistent about doing the practices at the end of the chapters and having all your materials ready. It is important to stop any excuses such as, "I just couldn't do it because I didn't feel good" or "I had an important meeting," "I forgot," "I'm depressed," "I didn't have enough time" and so forth.

My goal as your coach is to expect excellence, to bring out the very best in you. I am focused on your strengths and abilities, not on weaknesses. That's what it takes for success. Let yourself pause and take serious inventory. Stop and ask whether you are fully showing up for yourself in this program. I want you to be vigilant and mindful not to recycle self-defeating thoughts and patterns. Stop them immediately and replace them with your new FFF thoughts.

You are accountable for your thinking and internal dialogue. If you are not ready to be totally mindful and serious about what thoughts you engage, you should stop this program now. For you must develop an impenetrable focus in order to really change the subatomic particles of your body. You will be completely closing the portal that creates any mental connection between food and weight gain. You can do this, but it does take commitment.

During the healing, your own *Inner Adult* will also be coaching you. A coach's job is similar to that of a parent. Parents are required to attend to a child or baby no matter what else is going on. Children don't care if you are depressed or if your life is falling apart or you have to move. You are still required to meet their needs. You are expected to feed them, change them and so on, no matter what. In this same way, it is important to show up and do the necessary things for this program.

In Conclusion

The wisdom being imparted to you in this chapter is similar to doing a spiritual practice. It is asking for great mindfulness and alertness from your Warrioress so that no sabotaging thoughts sneak into your mind. *Taking a stand* is like doing a meditation. You must keep bringing yourself back to the stillness within (the FFF Mastery Keys). No matter what discomfort or thoughts come into your mind, body or emotions, your job is to not get distracted. Let mind chatter travel right through—like a flock of seagulls flying over you at the ocean. *Observe and just let them pass by.* Remembering the principles is like continually pressing a return button back to your center starting point.

Emmett Fox, in *Power Through Constructive Thinking*, speaks about what to do if your focus gets interrupted. He says that the problem is not really that you may be hearing destructive thoughts. Just hearing a negative thought will not hurt you. He likened this to the situation where a burning cinder falls on you. If you quickly wipe away the cinder, no harm is done. Likewise, if you do not dwell on negative thoughts passing through your mind, all is well. However, if you mull them over, they begin to burn a hole.

In a sense, it is not a food diet you will need, but a mental diet. So when you do your 2-Week Healing, remember that if you hear or see a sabotaging thought, such as "That ice cream is going to make you fat," just brush it off.

The practice session that follows provides many practical tools and techniques to ward off destructive thinking. This will help you hold an impeccable stand. You will go through important exercises and write out a meditation and healing to read every day. Spend as much time as you need to embody the knowledge before you go into the Ceremony and 2-Week Healing, which is described in the next chapter.

PRACTICE SESSION 8

Visual Aid: On a piece of paper, write the following key words and place them as a visual reminder in front of you. For groups, place the paper in the center of the circle. For this chapter, the sign will say:

~ Commitment ~
(to hold a focus or a stand long enough to change your body)

1. Opening Attunement (see sample on p. 13 or p. 14)

If you so desire, light a candle to mark the opening of the session. I recommend that you play the subliminal *Freedom From Food* CD quietly in the background during the attunement.

2. Check-In (2–3 Minutes)

For Individuals: Write a page or more in your journal as a check-in with yourself. Next, review the question that follows.

For Groups: Allow a 2–3-minute check-in, where you tell a little bit about yourself and address the following question. Also, please share what has been working for you this week to change your thinking about food. (Remember to pass the talking piece and use a timer.)

• What have you learned from the movie *A Beautiful Mind* about blocking out sabotaging voices?

3. 10-Minute Sharing

For Individuals: First read the following visualization and then write in your journal what comes up for you.

For Groups: This is a special time for one person (per session) to tell a personal story. It will allow you to get to know each person better. A lot of healing takes place by telling your story in the circle and having other people witness, support and deeply listen to you in a safe place. You need share only that which you feel comfortable to reveal. To begin, the leader can read the following visualization to the person whose turn it is. This will help you get in touch with what you would like to share.

Suggested Visualization to Assist the Sharing

I ask you to take a moment and close your eyes and connect with your heart. Now, I would like you to begin to follow the path that leads to your tears, pain, fear or any other emotion that connects you to your wound around food or weight (pause). Allow the important moments and events to come up (pause). Put an imaginary mirror up and look into it—not a physical look but an emotional one. What was your heart feeling then? What expression is on your face (pause)? Take a moment and let any other relevant scenes or feelings arise (pause). When you are ready, slowly open your eyes. If you are in a group, share your experience.

4. Appreciations

For Individuals: This is a good time to write down three appreciations of yourself—something about your essence. See the examples that follow.

For Groups: Three people from the group can give brief appreciations for the person who has just spoken. An appreciation should be something about one's essence—what you notice about that person. An appreciation should not give advice or include an explanation about how the person's story relates to your story. These are examples of the kinds of appreciations you might offer:

I love your courage and the way you speak up for yourself.
I appreciate how you protect your Inner Child.
I think you are radiant, and I love your smile.

5. Break

6. Share Your Homework (Saboteurs)

For Individuals: Reread your homework, in which you named and described your Inner Saboteur. Write in your journal any additional thoughts you have on the topic.

For Groups: Go around the circle and, one by one, read your homework paper, in which you named and described your Inner Saboteur. (The timekeeper should allow 2–3 minutes per person.)

7. Preparation for Taking Your 2-Week Stand

For Individuals: Practice the following exercises and write down your insights in your journal.

For Groups: Practice the following exercises and then share your experiences. You may want to choose one person to read the exercises aloud to the group.

a. Physiology of Taking a Stand. Physiology is important in creating a stand. In my experience, people feel stronger, more empowered and more alert when they are sitting straight. Their peripheral vision is open, and they are more watchful for both inner and outer sabotaging voices.

Exercise: To begin, sit slouched over and observe how you feel emotionally. Hold this posture for a minute. Next, put your shoulders back and sit up. Hold this posture for a minute. Observe how emotionally different you feel while sitting this way. Write your observations in your journal. (When you are doing your 2-Week Healing, straighten up if you feel your Inner Saboteurs are getting the best of you, wreaking havoc on your mind.)

b. Eye Focus. Go to the section in this chapter called Holding a Focus and do the exercise.

c. Blocking the Stomach Area. To block outside negative voices and mass consciousness beliefs about dieting, you must develop impenetrable boundaries around your stomach area, where the effects of sabotaging thoughts commonly enter. The following exercises will help you develop skills to achieve this protection.

Exercise 1: Picture an invisible shield around your stomach area or simply place your hands over it as a symbol of protection. Pause now and create the image of your choice.

Exercise 2: Picture someone throwing a punch at your stomach right now. Feel the way the muscles tighten to protect you from the blow. Make sure to release the block by exhaling when you no longer need it. Use this same response of tightening your stomach anytime you feel a sabotaging thought coming from others or your own internal voice. Practice the tightening process for quick, temporary help.

For Individuals: In your journal, write about what you have observed from the preceding exercise.

For Groups: Share what you have observed from the stomach block exercises. Form pairs and practice different stomach blocks. When you practice throwing a punch into the stomach, swing so that the punch does not really land. (Pretending to punch will create the necessary effect.) Then ask the person to report what muscles or sensations she tightened in response.

d. Moving Consciousness at Will. You can control where you put your attention rather than being the victim of old thoughts. You do have the power to keep your consciousness on the FFF principles when you are taking your stand. Energy flows where your attention goes. Practice your focus by doing the following visualization:

For Individuals: Read the visualization. In your journal, write about your experience.

For Groups: Choose one person to read this aloud to the others, who will close their eyes while sitting or lying down. Have your journal and a pen ready to write your observations. When you are finished, share your insights with the group.

Visualization

(Practice moving your focus around your body.)

First, visualize your energy in the back of your eyes. Bring your focus there (pause). Now, move your energy and focus to your left ear and be aware of any sensations (pause). Now, move your attention behind your bellybutton (pause). Move your attention to your right big toe and feel the sensation). Now, move your attention inside your heart area. Next, place your attention on your throat area (pause). Move your attention to your third eye, to the point between your eyebrows (pause). Finally, move your focus to the crown of your head and then to about 4–6 inches above your head. Good! Remember to move your consciousness to your upper areas (third eye, crown or higher) if negative thoughts start to bombard you during your stand.

8. Helpful Hint Tools List

The following list of helpful tools will support you during your 2-Week Healing process. Use it when you are feeling stuck or just need reinforcement. These tools are especially useful when sabotaging thoughts of doubt and failure are mentally attacking you. Keep this list where you can refer to it every day and take it along when you go out.

Part I—Read Aloud the List:

1. Remember that full is not fat and bloat is not fat. Trust your body to eliminate what it does not need.

2. Read over your notes on the Mastery Keys.

3. Listen to the *Freedom From Food* CD.

4. Practice tuning out any sabotaging voice that tries to enter. Act like this voice is an unwelcome, boring friend. Remember how you tune out people who just talk on and on and never really want to hear what you have to say. You may nod your head, but you are not listening to their words. Try it out. This is what children often do to adults when they do not feel like listening to them. For example, if people are talking about diets, you could tune them out by thinking about one of your favorite places in nature and picturing yourself there. Another option is to pretend they are speaking a foreign language you don't understand.

5. Cancel and replace unwanted thoughts with ideas that support you in this FFF process.

6. Think of your metabolism as being hungry critters that are eating up fat cells.

7. Put affirmations all around your house and say them repeatedly.

8. Visualize yourself taking in food and releasing it like air, knowing your body will keep only what it needs.

9. Tap the Karate Chop Point on your hand. You can say prepared phrases (see Chapter 7) silently to yourself or just tap the point.

10. *For Groups:* Call a friend for support and ask her to remind you of the Mastery Keys or any reinforcing thoughts from the program (doubts or negative thoughts are *not* to be exchanged at this time).

11. Sing a song, such as "Mary Had a Little Lamb," to block out what the negative voices are saying. Another alternative is to think like a child who does not want to listen and make a noise or soft hum to tune out someone.

12. See or feel unwelcome thoughts as rubber balls bouncing off your stomach. As a child, I remember saying, "I'm rubber, and you're glue. Everything you say bounces off me and sticks to you."

13. Remember the woman in the Olympics. Simulate how she keeps a laser-like focus on the balance beam by blurring out unwanted comments from the outside and by staying focused on what she is doing. This includes staying out of emotions or other things that may take your attention off course.

14. Picture an invisible shield around your stomach area or simply place your hands over it as a symbol of protection.

15. Focus up and keep your shoulders back.

16. Recall the expression "Fake it 'til you make it!"

17. See your body like a glass of champagne and excess bubbles (weight, food, energy) are rising off you.

18. Turn uncomfortable feelings and thoughts over to your Warrioress or Higher Self. Ask these wise parts of your personality to handle anything that is overwhelming. (Write down your worries, place the paper in a container and let it go. Trust that your problems will be handled.)

19. Be hyper-alert about the thoughts you entertain. Let into your consciousness only beneficial ideas from other people and the media.

20. Look at the pictures you created from magazines, where you

superimposed your face onto a magazine picture of your desired body.

21. Think of a sabotaging thought merely as a burning cinder that is flying onto your clothes. Remember, it burns a hole only if you give it time to stay there. So quickly brush it off and replace it with a positive thought.

Part II—Practice Eating While Using the Helpful Hint Tools

Exercise: Set up a few kinds of foods in front of you that are high in calories or scary for you to eat.

For Individuals:

a. Allow yourself to get prepared before you start to eat. You are going to have an interaction with three internal parts of yourself—a positive voice, a negative voice, and a listening part. Get prepared by doing the following:

• Sit straight, shoulders back and keep your focus up or straight ahead.

• Stay alert.

• Be ready to ward off any sabotaging thoughts that try to slip in. Think of yourself as a tiger, alert to invaders that might enter your space. Pull in your stomach and picture a shield of protection around it (Blocking the Stomach Area in section 7c. of the practice session, this chapter).

• Put the list of *Helpful Hint Tools* in front of you. Choose one item to practice while you are eating.

b. Begin to eat the food in front of you. First, as you are chewing, use your positive voice to remind yourself of two reasons why food does not make you gain weight. For example, think that food is only mindless energy without a brain or intention. It has no power to make you do anything. Think about the food going into your body and then being released automatically if there is excess.

c. Next, the negative voice will add something such as, "One moment on the lips, forever on your hips." After hearing the negative thought, remind yourself of the two positive reasons that food will not affect your weight to counteract the negative input. Pick something from the list of Helpful Hints Tools to help you fight off the negativity. Continue to eat while you practice different strategies and remember the ones that are most effective. Write them in your journal.

d. Keep repeating the exercise until you feel that you are winning the battle and are confident about blocking out sabotaging voices. Journal your experience.

Note: When you are out socializing, remind yourself that you can change the subject, walk away, say that you need to go to the restroom or assert that you are tired of listening to people talk about diets or weight. Refer to your Helpful Hint Tools for assistance.

For Groups:

a. Break up into groups of four. In the groups, two people will speak positive statements while the third person offers negative ones. The fourth person will eat while listening to the statements being spoken by the others. The challenge for the fourth person is to listen only to the positive voices that are reinforcing the FFF principles. She uses the *Helpful Hint Tools* to help ward off the negative voice. Each person in the group should have the opportunity to be the fourth person.

b. Allow yourself to get prepared before you begin by doing the following:

• Sit up, with shoulders back and your focus up or straight ahead.

• Stay alert.

• Be ready to ward off sabotaging thoughts that try to slip in. Think of yourself as a tiger, alert to invaders that might enter your space. When someone is speaking to you, decide if you want to hear what the person is saying. If not, use the Helpful Hint Tools to end the conversation.

• Pull in your stomach and picture a protective shield around it. (Review Blocking the Stomach Area in this practice session.)

Put the list of Helpful Hint Tools in front of you. Choose one of them to practice while you are eating.

c. Begin to eat. As you are chewing, the two positive speakers will talk first. Some examples of positive input are: "Food is only mindless energy without a brain or intention," "Food has no power to make you do anything" and "As you are eating, your body takes what it needs automatically and releases anything that is toxic or unhealthy." It is important to have this positive reinforcement flowing before you are challenged by conflicting voices.

d. The person with the negative voice then adds something such as, "One moment on the lips, forever on your hips." Now, the two positive speakers will again state that food will not affect your weight. Make sure the speakers do not bombard the listener by talking all at once. The fourth person, who is listening to these positive and negative voices, must stay focused on the positive. Continue to eat and practice different strategies from the Helpful Hint Tools list. Make a note of which items empower you the most so you can use them again when in need.

e. Keep practicing until you feel you are winning the battle and are confident about blocking out sabotaging voices. In your journal, write about your experience.

f. Next, each person in the group will do the exercise quietly alone and practice fighting her own sabotaging voices. Then share the experience with the group. If anyone has trouble, other people in the group can be of help.

Note: During the 2 weeks, when you are out socializing, remember you can change the subject, walk away, say you need to go to the restroom, assert that you are tired of listening to people talk about diets or weight and so on.

9. Naming Your Warrioress

This exercise allows you to get in touch with the Warrioress inside. She is the empowered, strong part that will get you through the 2-Week Healing process. Write a 1–2 page paper describing this part of yourself. For examples, see Warrioress section in this chapter. Share the paper with the group if you are in one.

10. Preparing Your Meditation for the 2-Week Healing

What follows is an example of a completed meditation. It is a combination of the two parts you will create next. The purpose of the meditation is to remind your subconscious and conscious mind of the FFF principles. You will state your intention about no longer gaining weight from food and recall the times in your life when you could eat what you wanted without putting on extra pounds. This meditation will continually bring into your awareness you body's innate intelligence to eliminate all unneeded food. It will create a road map, informing the subatomic particles of your body how to rearrange themselves.

Note: Do not start reading your daily meditation until after the Ceremony of Empowerment to preserve the potency. Trust the process!! (In the meditation, I am always referring to people in general without special medical conditions.)

a. Example of the Completed Meditation:

I know that food does not make me fat because I remember going to my aunt's holiday dinners when I was 10 years old and eating turkey, mashed potatoes, green beans, yams, fruit, pumpkin pie with whipped cream, birthday cake, carrots and biscuits with butter and gravy, and I did not gain weight. At 16, I remember going to my friend Steve's with Kathy and eating bags of candy corn, ice cream, lots of cookies and a bag of chocolate covered candies, and I did not gain weight. I remember when I was 5, my brother and I used to race and see how many pancakes we could eat, and I ate seven pancakes with tons of butter and syrup, and I did not gain weight. When I was 14, I remember going to a party and eating chocolate cake with chocolate frosting, cookies, rocky road and vanilla homemade ice cream, soda, punch and a candy bar, and I did not gain weight. Therefore, I know that it is not the food that makes me fat.

I also know that food does not make people fat because I remember my friend John, who drinks soda and eats lots of Mexican food with rice, drinks beer and finishes with an ice cream sundae. He does not gain weight, and I have seen him eat this way a lot. I also have a friend, Sue, who I have seen eat candy bars, ice cream, pasta, garlic bread, sour cream, salad and lots of potato chips and dip for starters, and she did not gain weight. She is thin and eats like this a lot. Therefore, I know that it is not an absolute truth that food makes people fat, for if it were an absolute truth, it must be true for all, and I know some people who are not affected in this way by food.

From the examples I have given as proof, I know that it is not food that makes me fat, for there have been many times that I have eaten huge amounts of food and not gained weight. I also know that food cannot make me fat, for I have mentioned some people who are skinny and eat whatever they want. Therefore, I conclude that it is not an absolute truth that food can make me fat, because if it were a truth for one person, it would have to be true for all.

I know that food of any kind is merely matter or effect and has no power over me. Since Mind is the only Cause, I know that it is only my mental thoughts that can cause bodily effects. I am totally confident that it is not the amount of food, how much food, the times I eat food or the kinds of foods that make me fat. Food cannot cause me to do anything. Food is neutral, nonintentional, mindless energy that has no power over me.

Therefore, I will eat whatever I want, eat as much as I want and not gain weight. I will weigh myself in 2 weeks from when I started, and I will not have gained any weight. I will never gain weight again, no matter how many days I eat consistently. I am absolutely sure that food does not affect my weight.

I know this is so,
So it is,
Expect a Miracle!!!
Love,
_____(sign your name)

b. Now You Are Ready to Write Your Own Meditation. To start this process of creating your own version of the above meditation, you need to gather some past memories. You most likely have had times in your life, before you took this course, when you ate whatever you wanted, as much as you wanted, and did not gain weight. Maybe it was as a child, an adolescent, or at a time in your life when you were on a vacation or when you were in love. You were probably not even thinking much about food during these times. (Take a few moments and make notations of your recollections. You can add these to your meditation.)

At the very least, you were not fat when you came out of the womb. Even if a person has normal baby fat at birth, it generally goes away. However, weight problems can develop if you received negative programming that became embedded in your conscious or unconscious mind, or if you had a medical problem.

The following visualization will assist you in retrieving some positive childhood memories about times you ate and did not gain weight. There is also a segment in which you will try to remember five examples of other people who could eat a lot and not put on extra pounds. You will then use all of the collected memories to create the first part of your daily meditation. The purpose of recalling these times is to reawaken your conscious mind to the idea that you already know somewhere in your psyche how to eat and not gain weight.

Exercise: Visualization to Get Examples for Your Meditation

For Individuals: Read the visualization below. In your journal, write about your experience.

For Groups: Choose one person to read this aloud to the rest of the group while they are sitting or lying down with eyes closed. Have your journal and pen ready to write your observations. When you are finished, share your answers with the group.

Visualization

I invite you to take some deep breaths, breathing all the way in and holding it and then letting out all the air. Continue breathing at your own pace. Now, allow yourself to go back in time to places, situations and people from your past. You can go back and remember things that you have not thought about for a long while. Just allow yourself to travel back to a time before you began gaining weight...a time when you remember eating and being thin (long pause).

Begin by first picturing the table where you ate meals as a child. Take a look around and see what food was on the table and what people were present (pause). Try to remember favorite meals your mom, relatives or others would make (pause). What were your favorite foods or snacks? Recall the smells. Picture the food you ate in detail. See the amounts you ate and exactly what you ate. Maybe you consumed pancake breakfasts until you were stuffed but did not gain weight. Maybe you and your friends sometimes ate things such as white bread, cinnamon toast, cookies, candy and ice cream and you did not gain weight. Maybe you remember big holiday dinners where you ate turkey, mashed potatoes, stuffing, pie and so forth. You might have been full, but you did not gain weight. Your body just seemed to eliminate any excess food by the next day. Give yourself time to remember (long pause).

Next, I would like you to think of other people who could eat whatever they wanted and were always thin. For example, think about aunts, uncles, cousins, grandparents, parents, teachers, friends and boyfriends and what you observed them eating (long pause).

Now, take a deep breath in and gently come back into the room. Begin to write in detail the examples you remembered.

c. Now Write out the First Part of Your Meditation. The following is an example of how to write your first two paragraphs. Use the exact format with your own examples, gathered from the above visualization, and include all the parts that are underlined without changing them:

Creating the First Part:

I know that food does not make me fat because I remember going to my aunt's holiday dinners when I was 10 years old and eating turkey, mashed potatoes, green beans, yams, fruit, pumpkin pie with whipped cream, birthday cake, carrots and biscuits with butter and gravy, and I did not gain weight. When I was 16, I remember going to my friend Steve's with Kathy and eating bags of candy corn, ice cream, lots of cookies and a bag of chocolate covered candies, and I did not gain weight. I remember when I was 5, my brother and I used to race and see how many pancakes we could eat, and I ate seven pancakes with tons of butter and syrup, and I did not gain weight. When I was 14, I remember going to a party and eating chocolate cake with chocolate frosting, cookies, rocky road and vanilla homemade ice cream, coke and punch and a candy bar, and I did not gain weight. (You can add two more examples.) Therefore, I know that it is not food that makes me fat.

I also know that food does not make people fat because I remember my friend John who drinks soda and eats lots of Mexican food with rice, drinks beers and finishes with an ice cream sundae. He does not gain weight, and I have seen him eat this way a lot. I also have a friend, Sue, who I have seen eating candy bars, ice cream, lots of pasta, garlic bread, sour cream, salad and lots of potato chips and dip to begin with, and she does not gain weight. She is thin and eats like this a lot. (Add some more examples like this.) Therefore, I know it is not an absolute truth that food makes a person fat, for if it were an absolute truth, it must be true for all, and I know that these people I've just mentioned are not affected in this way by food.

d. Now Write out the Last Part of Your Meditation. You may use the following three paragraphs exactly as they are or you can add some sentences taken from this course to create the first two paragraphs of this last part. However, keep the third paragraph as it is.

For Groups: If you add things to the following example, make a copy for everyone else in the group. It is good to have as many ideas as possible.

Creating the Last Part:

From the examples I have given as proof, I know that it is <u>not</u> food that makes me fat, for there have been many times that I have eaten huge amounts of food and not gained weight. I also know that food cannot make me fat, for I have mentioned some people who are skinny and eat whatever they want. Therefore, I <u>conclude</u> that it is <u>not an absolute</u> truth that food can make me fat, because if it were an absolute truth for one *person, it would have to be true for all.*

I know that food of any kind is merely matter or effect and has <u>no power over me</u>. Since Mind is the <u>only Cause</u>, I know that it is <u>only my mental thoughts</u> that can cause bodily effects. I am <u>totally confident</u> that it is not the amount of food, how much food, the times I eat food or the kinds of foods that make me fat. Food <u>cannot cause</u> me to do anything. Food is neutral, nonintentional, mindless energy that has no power over me.

Therefore, I <u>will</u> eat whatever I want, eat as much as I want and not gain weight. I will weigh myself in 2 weeks from when I started, and I will not have gained any weight. I will <u>never gain weight again.</u> No matter how many days I eat consistently. I am <u>absolutely sure that food does not affect my weight.</u>

I know this is so,

So it is,

Expect a Miracle!!!

Love,

_____*(sign your name)*

e. Put Together the Two Parts to Create Your Completed Meditation. The final step in writing out your meditation is to put together the two parts you have created. Simply join the two paragraphs you wrote in the previous section, called "Creating the First Part" with the three paragraphs you wrote in the previous section, called "Creating the Last Part." You then will have a completed meditation to use for your 2-Week Healing.

Note: Women planning to get pregnant might consider the following. When I wrote out my meditation, I knew I wanted to have a baby in the future. Therefore, I added the following words to the end of my meditation: "If I get pregnant, I will gain the perfect amount that my baby needs for its health, and all unneeded, excess weight will come off easily after I give birth."

11. A List of Things to Bring to the Ceremony

The Ceremony of Empowerment takes place next week instead

of your normal practice.

For Individuals: The following items are mandatory for you to prepare and bring to the Ceremony.

For Groups: The following items are mandatory for you to prepare and bring to the Ceremony. If you forget any of these, you will need to go back home and get them. Accountability is essential for you as a Warrioress. It is necessary to show up impeccably, 100 percent for yourself with no excuses.

a. Create an outfit that expresses the Warrioress part of you and wear it during the Ceremony. Bring a piece of paper with your Warrioress name written on it. You will place this in front of you.

b. Bring a paper that tells about times in your life when you already have taken a stand successfully (for example, always getting a parking place, never getting sick, etc.).

c. From the following script, create an audiotape with the title Practice Eating at the Ceremony.

For Individuals: Prepare the tape now to play for yourself at the Ceremony.

For Groups: Choose one person to make the tape for the Ceremony.

Script: Practice Eating at the Ceremony

Focus on the thing at this table setting that brings you to <u>the highest thought about food</u> (pause). Begin eating as you do this. Your highest thought may be a color that reminds you of the life force or energy of a particular food, a candle that reminds you that food is light energy not dense matter, some flowers that remind you of the beauty of your body in perfect proportion and so on (pause awhile…write in your journal what came up for you…or share with the group, if you are in one).

Now, continue eating while <u>focusing on your senses</u>. First touch the food and feel the texture. Then take a bite and allow your taste buds to awaken to various flavors while you remember that all food is just harmless energy here to enjoy. Next, allow the smells to trigger one of your highest thoughts about food. As you begin chewing, allow the sounds to trig-

ger the awareness that your body is starting to break down the food. Feel the sensations as you chew. Realize that your only job in the process is to chew up the food. The moment you swallow, you must let go and begin to trust your body to do its job. Remember its innate intelligence is to take in what is needed and eliminate the rest (pause awhile...write in your journal what came up for you...or share with the group, if you are in one).

Next, as you are eating, allow yourself to <u>freely associate</u> from one thought to the next about the truths and principles you have studied. For example, in the following sequence, you might think about food like this:

...If you get a cut, your body always creates antibodies to heal itself. This might lead you to think about another way your body heals itself by eliminating all excess food that is not needed or toxic. You then might freely associate to thoughts about your connection to nature and how flowers and undomesticated animals don't diet and yet they always have a perfect proportion...(pause awhile...write in your journal what came up for you...or share with the group, if you are in one).

Now, practice eating while using the power of your <u>will</u> to disarm any saboteurs. Get into your Warrioress stance and will them away by keeping your thoughts vigilantly on the FFF principles about food. Picture yourself walking a tightrope while focused on the Mastery Keys, not losing your balance from listening to negative thoughts. Remember the scenes in the movie, A Beautiful Mind. *Use the Helpful Hints Tools to assist you. Make sure you are in your Warrioress stand with shoulders back, spine straight, mind alert and stomach area tightened or shielded in some way (pause awhile...write in your journal what came up for you...or share with the group, if you are in one).*

d. Bring a long-lasting candle if you can find one. This will also be used as a focal point during your 2-Week Healing.

e. It is nice to bring flowers and an object that symbolizes your own personal power.

f. Bring different foods that are binge foods or scary foods for you to practice eating while you fight sabotaging thoughts (such as candy, french fries, cheese, nuts, bread, ice cream, cakes, pizza, etc.).

g. Bring your list of Helpful Hint Tools to use while taking your stand.

h. Record a tape using the script, called Ending Visualization, which can be found in Chapter 9. If you can locate the theme song from *Chariots of Fire*, bring it to play softly in the background.

For Individuals: Prepare the tape now and play it at the Ceremony.

For Groups: Choose one person to make the tape and bring a tape recorder to the Ceremony.

i. Bring your completed Healing Meditation.

Note: Allot more than the usual amount of time for next week's Ceremony. For groups, it could take 4–5 hours or more to complete.

12. Homework

This week, your homework assignment is to do the following:

a. Review the Mastery Keys and other principles as presented in past chapters. Write a few sentences on each one of the following:

- Diets Don't Work
- First Mastery Key—The Body Heals Itself
- Second Mastery Key—Mind Creates Matter
- Third Mastery Key—Emotions Affect Your Body
- Fourth Mastery Key—Food Is Energy
- Saboteurs

b. Make preparations for the Ceremony of Empowerment.

Reminder for groups: Choose a new leader for next week.

9. Appreciation

For Individuals: Write a few sentences in your journal about what most moved or inspired you in this chapter.

For Groups: Go around the circle. Speak about what most moved and inspired you in the meeting today.

10. Closing Attunement (see sample on p. 13 or p. 14)

PART IV

DEMONSTRATION AND
TRANSFORMATION

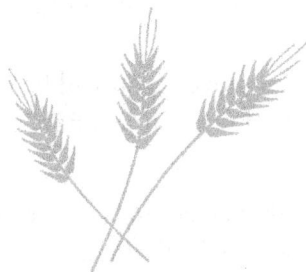

NINE

CEREMONY OF EMPOWERMENT FOLLOWED BY THE 2-WEEK HEALING

In every contest, there comes a moment that defines winning from losing. The true warrior understands and seizes that moment by giving an effort so intensive and so intuitive that it could only be called one from the heart.

—Pat Riley

The Wise Woman Speaks

Sitting in a sacred area in the forest surrounded with beautiful flowers, the Wise Woman is ready to assist your transition into the next passage. Wearing an exquisitely jeweled ceremonial robe, she stands straight, holding an eagle feather, with her shoulders back and her head held high. Exuding the magnificence, power and alertness of a tiger, she begins to speak:

~

You have arrived at a major transformational point in this journey. It is now time for you to go through the Ceremony of Empowerment, the gateway of preparation that precedes the 2-Week Healing.

The Warrioress inside of you will ultimately get you through this test of fire, which is an initiation to remove the veils that cloud you from knowing how to keep your body temple in harmony.

Once those clouds are removed, you will be able to complete the 2-Week Healing and find yourself in a new state of consciousness about food.

I am calling for your 100 percent focus. I am asking for your word to make a stand for the new FFF principles, with no excuses now. This has the potential to change your relationship with food for the rest of your life if, and only if, you are committed to hold the new consciousness. There will be no going back. Are you ready?

———

In this chapter, you will become familiar with the Ceremony of Empowerment and the 2-Week Healing. The actual instructions and complete guidelines will be given to you in the practice sessions that follow.

Ceremony of Empowerment

The Ceremony is most empowering when it is held in an atmosphere of integrity, safety and the sacred. In this clear space, you focus your intentions and root them deeply into your mind and emotions. Supported by a fertile, receptive environment, your thoughts will easily drop in and begin to grow. This sets in motion the desired currents of energy to ripple through your cells on their way to manifestation. Take a moment and picture in your mind the kind of environment that will create this nourishing experience.

During the Ceremony, you are going to be practicing different exercises. Of course, part of this will be eating and dealing with Saboteurs that try to shatter the coherency of your stand. The challenge is to align your mind and body in a refrain of pure laser-like intention, enabling you to shift your thoughts out of any remaining inertia and victimization around food. To do this, you create a continuous flow of the new FFF ideas.

You support this new mindset by carefully choosing conversations and words that carry the frequency of your new beliefs. For example, you test yourself with different foods such as bread and butter, cookies, pecans, avocados—whatever has been on your list of fattening foods. Then, as your Saboteurs try to get you off track, bringing up familiar phrases such as "One moment on the lips, forever on your hips," you counteract their imposter voices with truths from the program. You might say, "I now know that all food is energy, and it has no power to make me gain weight. It is my mind that directs what the energy does. Therefore, I am affirming right now that my body will take what it needs from this food and release the rest." Reinforce your words by creating a visual image and connect with any feelings this elicits in your body.

Readiness Check

After practicing various exercises during the Ceremony to reinforce all that you have learned, you will take an assessment of how prepared you feel to begin the 2-Week Healing that starts the following day. In this assessment, you will need to put to test any reason not to show up for the program. Ask yourself, "If this were my night to perform at the Olympics, would any of my excuses be valid?"

Remember, it is common for Saboteurs to come at you the strongest just before you are ready to make a significant change. They will distract you by pulling your attention off the FFF focus and onto worrying about relationships, business and so forth. The Saboteurs that have helped you survive until now are well aware that your success will be the end of them. They can put up a fight to see how determined you really are to make this shift.

Here are some questions to ask yourself:

• Am I ready to call forth all of my strength, courage, self-esteem and ability to draw boundaries and say "No" when it is appropriate?

• Am I ready to take back all of my energy and power and put it into the 2-week healing process?

• Am I ready to nurture and love myself deeply and commit to the FFF principles?

- Am I ready to make this stand a No. 1 priority in my life?

Next, you pick a number from 1 to 10 to assess how ready you actually feel. The following is an example of how one participant in the program did this:

~

The most poignant moment of the evening for me was when Patricia asked, "Who is committed? Where are you on a scale of 1–10?" I scanned my mind and asked myself the question. In that moment, I realized that my mind was the only thing that could hold me back from being a 10. So I made a choice. I chose 10.

My inner dialogue took a fraction of a second: "It's now or never. Shit or get off the pot. There are all these supportive people telling me that I can do this and that the process is a truth. What would possibly hold me back from believing in it? I've been replaying my internal tapes of self-defeating thoughts for too long. They're boring. I don't want to go there anymore. I choose not to go there anymore. I CHOOSE TO BELIEVE THAT I CAN EAT WHATEVER I WANT AND NOT GAIN WEIGHT."

This was definitely a Warrioress stance, and I felt my Warrioress step forward. She was in me and I "knew"—and I said, "Yes, count me in," with conviction in my heart.

I know that I can do this. I won't deprive myself of this freedom. I have wanted to believe something like this [the principles of Freedom From Food] for ages, and here is a teacher and a time in my life to embrace and live these principles. I want to feel comfortable in my clothes. I want to enjoy my relationship with food. I want to be PERFECTLY PROPORTIONED.

—Participant

~

In the last part of the Ceremony, if you feel you are prepared, your Higher Self or the group will witness you making your commitment to proceed with the stand. Holding a stand like this one is something people rarely, if ever, do for themselves. The rewards and the self-empowerment are transformational and applicable to so many areas of your life. You are rewriting the movie. I believe you are worth it. I hope you do!

The 2-Week Healing

The morning after the Ceremony of Empowerment, you begin the 2-Week Healing. This is a period of time in which you demonstrate what you have learned about using your mind to affect your body. In a sense, you are going into the alchemical laboratory where you combine your mind, emotions and intention to rearrange the formless into form. You will be activating your new beliefs in order to receive the sacrament of this teaching. As your body systems begin to speed up and wake up, they can ignite a quickening fire to your metabolism, releasing what has been stagnant and stuck. Be prepared to burn away the old and welcome in the new.

The strength of your focus accelerates the change in your physical form and moves you from intellectual understanding into actual manifestation. Aligning in this way breaks the connection between what you eat and gaining weight. Afterward, there will be nothing to which negative fat thoughts can stick. Your healing will become a prayer of trust in your body's ability to seamlessly eliminate all that is toxic or unhealthy, which includes excess weight. The exhilarating outcome will be that you can eat whatever you want without putting on extra pounds.

The 2-Week Healing provides measurable, concrete evidence to evaluate your progress. You weigh yourself at the beginning and then at the end. This is your feedback device to determine the strength of your body/mind connection and remove any guesswork about whether you have gained weight or not. I think you will be wonderfully surprised at your ability to affect the flow in your body. Often people are afraid at this point and wonder if they can do it. What I have found is that most people are able to hold their stand and are tremendously successful.

You can let go to the natural rhythm—the ebb and flow—of ingesting, digesting and eliminating with the same ease as inhaling and exhaling. Your only job in the process is to enjoy as your taste buds awaken to the food. Chew it up and then the moment you swallow, let go and begin to trust your body to do its job of breaking down what you have eaten. Imagine doing this—taking in food, letting it go…taking in food, letting it go…

Although it is not the goal or the norm to lose a few pounds during the 2 weeks, some of my participants, without knowing when it happened, lost weight (or their size changed) during or even before they did the healing. They were not checking or trying to reduce. It just happened. Losing weight will be discussed in the next chapter.

Participants' Comments

(Here is what a few participants had to say about the 2-Week Healing)

Finally, it was time to do "The Healing." The point of the healing was to show us that indeed we were ready to eat whatever we want and not gain weight. We were told to weigh ourselves and for the next 14 days to eat as much as we desired and that we would weigh ourselves again in 2 weeks' time.

Luckily for me, I already knew how tricky the human mind could be, and so I was determined to go for it. What I mean by that is I knew that if I did not eat as much as I possibly could, if indeed after the 2 weeks I had not gained any weight, I would be thinking things such as if I had eaten more, I would have gained weight and so on.

So for the next 2 weeks, every day I ate a huge muffin for breakfast, a big lunch and dinner, pastries, chocolate and just about everything else I could get into myself. In those days, I was the type that could easily gain five pounds in a week with a diet like that. Two weeks later, I weighed in at exactly the same weight as 2 weeks previously!

—Participant

I remember being astounded with how much I ate that I didn't gain 20 pounds. I remember eating hamburgers, french fries and sundaes and not gaining weight. After that time, I exercised but not neurotically or compulsively, and I ate what I wanted. I would eat a lot at Thanksgiving or Christmas or parties and never gain weight. I found that my body when I didn't interfere would just balance out. I believe that the food will just dissolve in the ethers. You don't have to burn it off. It just goes away. I found you can even just lie in bed and it just dissolves. It's like air; it just goes in and goes out. I now understand that matter has no substance. Consciousness is the source of my freedom.

—Participant

I have felt incredibly focused all the way through these two weeks. Driving over to my friend's house to weigh myself this morning, I was excited. I felt sure of myself, sure of holding the stance. Then just before weighing myself I had a moment of panic. The thoughts came crowding in and I didn't listen to them, shut them out and got on the scale. It showed me that I had not gained weight. Instead I had lost four pounds! Power to the Angel of Food and Weight and Perfect Proportion.

—Participant

Thinland

During the months that follow, you will be creating the environment in consciousness that will allow you to make a quantum leap into a new paradigm around food and weight. As you hold to the principles in the 2-Week Healing, you will create a bridge to a different reality where you can take up residence permanently. I call this place Thinland.

In Thinland, people eat and do not gain weight, just like the thin people in your life (meaning those in their perfect proportion). Here there are no conversations about extra pounds, counting calories or restricted eating plans. People in this place expend their energy enjoying and living life. Exploring ways to evolve and become happier, they concentrate their thoughts and actions on increasing the quality of existence. Their lives are not about food and what the scale says but are more concerned with expressing individual gifts and passions. They come from a place of *deep* and *unquestioning knowing* that they can eat whatever they want and never gain weight. Can you think of anyone like this?

During the 2-Week Healing, you have a window of opportunity to relocate to Thinland. What happens during this period to permit such a change? Hugh Everett III, a pioneering physicist from Princeton University, has a theory about profound shifts that happen in life, causing us to move to a parallel possibility. According to Gregg Braden in *The Isaiah Effect*, Everett gives a name to the moments in time when the course of events may be altered. Everett called these windows of opportunity "choice points." A choice point occurs when conditions appear that create a path between the present course of events (such as food making you gain weight) and a new course leading to new outcomes (a thin person's reality). The choice point is like a bridge (in FFF, holding your stand for 2 weeks creates the bridge), making it possible to begin one path and change course to experience the outcome of a new path (where food no longer creates weight).

Visualization

(Use this Ending Visualization to activate the feeling of success in your body/mind during the Ceremony of Empowerment and the 2-Week Healing.)

Begin by taking three deep breaths, filling all the way up with air and holding it (at your own pace) and then exhaling all the air from your body (repeat)(pause). Now, bring your awareness to the crown of your head, open it like a skylight and let a golden energy begin to flow in. It fills your head with light and continues down to fill up your heart (take a deep breath in).

Now, allow an image of yourself to appear. Observe yourself carefully in detail. See the places on your body where you have been holding onto weight. Silently tell these parts of your body that they no longer need to store up calories (heat units of energy), because you are not hibernating. Your Adult Self is now willing to draw boundaries around you to create the safety you need. See the cells of your body receiving that message and releasing any kind of weight energy that you are holding.

Now, see yourself eating something that in the past would have been frightening to eat and weight producing. With your new way of thinking, however, you can see your body naturally releasing the excess food (heat units of energy). As you feel the food go through your body, say mentally, "I now release all unneeded food energy" (take a deep breath in).

See yourself getting on the scale to begin your 2-Week Healing. Then picture yourself eating anything you want during these 2 weeks. See all excess energy of food being eliminated automatically. Observe yourself not gaining weight no matter how much you eat. The excess food energy flows out of your body like an unobstructed stream.

Next, see yourself at the end of the 2 weeks, getting on the scale and observing that you have not gained weight. Create the feeling in your body of knowing that you can eat whatever you want, eat as much as you want and not put on extra pounds. In every cell, feel the sensation of your success. Let the feeling take over your whole being. Expand it even more. Feel and know that you have totally defused and disempowered food from ever making you gain weight again. Visualize yourself elated and strong as you celebrate the outcome of your 2-Week Healing. Now, take a deep breath in and release it. Slowly begin to bring your awareness back and observe your surroundings.

The Wise Woman Speaks

⁓

Having come this far, you have all the resources necessary to succeed. You have prepared and practiced all that you need to know. I am confident that you can do this next step. Stay focused, present and strong through this initiation, being mindful of all we have talked about. Your understanding of the Mastery Keys and how the body/mind works will be your strength and safety net. Remember, this is an energy world that is constantly fluctuating.

Further down the road, you will see a protected cabin where you can cocoon for 2 weeks while you are doing your healing. Refer to your Mastery Keys and the principles you have learned. This is the time where your form will be changing as the "imaginal cells" you have planted reach their point of transformation. Believe and trust in the laws of the unseen world that will begin to coagulate around the FFF ideas you hold.

Here, you can allow yourself to leap into the unknown. Your belief, trust and understanding will catch you and gently cushion your transition into Thinland. I will see you there. I wish you well until we see each other again.

⁓

You are now ready to begin the Ceremony of Empowerment, which will be followed by the 2-Week Healing.

PRACTICE SESSION 9

Ceremony of Empowerment Guidelines

For Individuals: The time for you to complete the Ceremony of Empowerment will vary. To begin the process, make sure you have all the required materials ready and in front of you.

For Groups: This meeting will take approximately 4–5 hours with no interruptions to complete. However, you may need to stay longer if someone requires more time. You must not proceed until everyone is totally committed, focused and ready to begin the 2-Week Healing the following morning. All members of the group must attend and have all of the materials with them before you start.

Visual Aid: Put the papers with the guiding words from all of the previous chapters in front of you

For Individuals: Set up a special place in your house. Honor yourself by beautifying and empowering the space in a way that feels comfortable.

For Groups: Set up a special place in one of your homes. As a group, honor yourselves by making the space beautiful and empowering.

List of Items to Place in Front of You

- The 2-Week Healing meditation you have written out

- A copy of the Helpful Hints Tools

- A name tag with the name of your female Warrioress on it

- A list of situations in which you are already successful in holding a stand and have a knowing that you can always achieve your desired outcome (for example, finding parking spaces, never getting sick and so on)

- Flowers for beauty, candles and some object that is empowering to you (optional)

- The Practice Eating at the Ceremony tape and Ending

Visualization tape placed in front of the leader along with a tape recorder (Keep your food in a separate area until instructed further)

1. Opening Attunement (see sample on p. 13 or p. 14)

If you so desire, light a candle to mark the opening of the session. I recommend that you play the subliminal *Freedom From Food* CD quietly in the background during the attunement.

2. Ceremony of Empowerment

Welcome Opening (Read aloud)

Welcome to the Ceremony of Empowerment! You have come a long way to get to this passage. This Ceremony is designed to give you the opportunity to evaluate for yourself whether you are indeed prepared to advance to the 2-Week Healing. You will be given many exercises and ways to assess your readiness. The material you will go over is the culmination of all of the concepts you have been learning. Therefore, most of the information and exercises will be a review from previous chapters.

If you have seriously done the practice sessions up to this point in the program, you most likely will find yourself ready to proceed. During this process, you will have a feeling of jumping into the unknown. Going forward will require trust in what you have learned. If you need to do more review or more work on yourself, it is perfectly OK. Give yourself the extra time.

Ceremony is a way to draw attention and energy to a time of completion and the beginning of a new phase in your life. It is the time for you to move to Thinland. To make that move, you will have the opportunity to finish up any old ways of thinking about food.

This Ceremony calls forth the female Warrioress in you. Fierce, strong and empowered, she holds impenetrable boundaries about what she believes and knows to be true. She is the part of you that ultimately will get you through this journey, this test of fire. This is the initiation to remove the veils of your mind that cloud you from knowing your full strength and how to keep your body temple in harmony.

For Groups: If you are ready to make this commitment to yourself and go through the Ceremony, please say your Warrioress name aloud.

About the Upcoming 2-Week Healing Process (Read aloud)

The morning following the Ceremony, you will begin the 2-Week Healing to prove that you can eat whatever you want, eat whenever you want and not gain weight.

You will hold this 2-week stand like a prayer of trust in your body's ability to automatically eliminate all that is not healthy (excess weight) or toxic to your system. It will be essential for you to replace any negative thought with your new ideas from the FFF program. This practice will inform the cells and subatomic particles of your body to rearrange in a way that food will no longer make you gain weight. You will need absolute attention and vigilance, like a person walking a tightrope. While eating, remind yourself that food is sacred and that Mother Earth has supplied it to sustain our lives as well as for us to enjoy.

3. Check-In (2–3 Minutes)

For Individuals: Write in your journal the things you are doing to reinforce your stand.

For Groups: Allow a 2–3-minute check-in where you speak about what you have been doing to reinforce your stand. Limit this check-in to positive responses only!!! (Remember to pass the talking piece and use a timer.)

4. Instructions for Beginning Your 2-Week Healing Process

Read the following instructions aloud in preparation for the 2-Week Healing, which starts tomorrow morning when you weigh in.

- The most important instruction is this: *Eat whatever you want, as much as you want and whenever you want!!!*

- Weigh yourself the first day only. Write down the time you stepped on the scale, the day and how much you weigh. Then put the scale away for 2 weeks and do not get on it for any reason!!! Getting on the scale just feeds your doubts.

• Read the meditation for 10 minutes daily. It may help to read it aloud. Put feeling behind the words as you say them. Read the meditation once, twice, three times or more until 10 minutes are up.

• It is helpful *not* to discuss this process with anyone until you have completed it. This conserves your energy so it is not diluted by having to explain or prove the validity of the program to others before you have successfully demonstrated it yourself. It will probably take several months before you feel strong in your new reality. Be protective and nurturing to yourself during this time.

• Keep your emotions on hold as much as possible during these 2 weeks. Your problems and emotions will be there afterward, right where you left them. Remember, if you focus down into your emotions, you are leaving an opening for the Saboteurs. Keep your energy up. Think of the Olympics and the women who compete on the balance beam. Remind yourself of their undivided attention as they performed. Walk away from any conversations that are not helpful. Make up an excuse to get away. Change any TV channels that interfere with what you are doing for these 2 weeks. (Review the list describing healthy instincts in Chapter 7.)

• If you desire, you can light a candle each day to start your meditation time and invite in your Higher Self or the Over-lighting Angel of Food and Weight. (It's great if you can find a long-lasting candle.)

• Do not look in the mirror to see how you are doing during these 2 weeks. Do not try on clothes that tell you how you are doing. Do not feel into your body to check. All of these are fatal moves of doubt. They are sabotaging moves that are no different than actually getting on a scale. Many of the participants found it helpful to cover up the mirrors in their house for 2 weeks or longer. Remember the saying "The watched pot never boils" (see Avoid the Mirror, 8c. in the Chapter 10 practice session).

• For 2 weeks only, I advise you not to exercise excessively. Many people have a body/mind link indicating that they must exercise to be thin. As I have stated, the trouble with this idea is that if you were too sick to be physically active, your body would most likely begin to gain weight in accordance with your belief system (see What About Exercise? in Chapter 3). Therefore, it is best to prove to yourself that whether you exercise or not, food does not make you gain weight.

• *For Groups:* Call the people in the group for support. Do not call them with your doubts. However, you can ask them to reinforce any of the FFF principles. The following are some suggestions of positive inquiries: "Will you remind me of why food can't make me fat?" "Will you share some things that are working for you during this healing?" "Will you speak to me of my body's natural ability to heal itself?"

• Make sure you are using the Helpful Hint Tools.

• Expect a miracle!!!

Note: In no way should you do anything that goes against what a doctor or other health professional has advised for your health!!! Do not test foods to which you are allergic or that you know would adversely affect your health in any way. You can eat whatever you want and still stay within the guidelines that a professional has laid out for you.

5. Instructions for Ending Your 2-Week Healing Process

• After 2 weeks, weigh in at the same time, at the same place and dressed in the same clothes you had on when you began.

• Remember, the sabotaging mind is tricky!! It will try to say things like, "Sure you weigh the same, but you had a sweater on when you first weighed yourself and now you don't. Also, you weighed in at the beginning at 11 am and now it's 8 am." This kind of sabotaging thinking wants to make you doubt your results. Because of the tricky mind, take away as many variables as possible when you weigh yourself again.

- After stepping on the scale, take a moment to acknowledge your success.

- Review and make some notes in your journal as to how much you ate and what you've just experienced. (I realize that some people may have even lost weight, although that is not the goal at this time.)

- Breathe in the miracle. Feel the power of your intention. Do not double-check yourself! Get on the scale once and then put it away for good!!!

- Reread Testimonials for 2-Week Healing in this chapter.

6. Helpful Hint Tools List

Read aloud the Helpful Hint Tools List and become familiar with these techniques (see the Chapter 8 practice session). For the following 2 weeks, keep them in the same place where you read your daily meditation. Also make a copy to carry around with you during the day.

7. Practice Eating Exercise

Now it is time in the Ceremony to play the tape called Practice Eating at the Ceremony, which you created from the Chapter 8 practice session. Before you begin, create a plate of the fabulously scrumptious food you have prepared for this occasion.

For Individuals: Now, play the tape. Write in your journal what comes up for you. The next exercise is to practice eating and using the Helpful Hint Tools. (Find the details of how to do this in the Chapter 8 practice session called Practice Eating and Using the Helpful Hint Tools.)

For Groups: Bring your plate of food back to your seat. Create a nice setting in the center of the circle with all of the extra food so that people can have seconds without getting up again. Now, play the tape to guide you through this exercise. Share your insights with the group. The next exercise is to practice eating and using the Helpful Hint Tools. (Find the details of how to do this in the Chapter 8 practice session called Practice Eating and Using the Helpful Hint Tools.)

8. Accountability and Readiness to Proceed to the 2-Week Healing

Part I. Assessing Your Readiness

This is the place in the Ceremony where you must take a deep, honest look into yourself, assessing whether you are ready to take a stand and commit to the new FFF thinking. Are you willing to put your problems and emotions on hold for 2 weeks while you focus completely on the Mastery Keys? Are you ready to place this healing and yourself as the No. 1 priority?

To begin assessing your readiness, read aloud the following message from the Wise Woman:

—

I want all parts of you here now. I call in your Warrioress, the ferocious tiger part of you that will stand up for your life. She is no longer willing to accept poison from Inner Saboteurs who want to keep you small, powerless, overweight and feeling insignificant. This is the part of you that is the empowered woman who is ready to fight for your well-being and draw boundaries. She is able to drop being a nice guy who allows others to walk over her. She is prepared to do whatever it takes to return to her perfectly proportioned body.

Now, I want you to visualize that I am looking you directly in the eyes. Picture both of us on a tightrope, facing each other. Feel how important it is for each of us not to lose our focus by letting in any doubts. Are you 100 percent ready to hold your balance and be totally aligned in thoughts and actions around the FFF principles?

It is necessary for you to shut off any part of your mind that wants to believe that you can't do this, any part that plays small. As if you were listening to the radio, turn the channel to the station or part of your personality that is accountable and strong. The one that has fed, clothed and found shelter for you no matter what has been going on. The one that has helped you through this FFF process and wants you to grow and thrive. You would not be alive if some part of you was not consistently helping you survive all the trials and tribulations of life. I am asking this Warrioress to come out now, empowered and in full strength for these 2 weeks. I believe in you. It is the time to reclaim yourself.

Are you ready to succeed? We are not in dress rehearsal anymore!!! This is not for the wishy-washy or faint of heart. This is for the trained, empowered Warrioress within.

Part II. Picking a Number to Indicate Your Readiness

Now it is time in the Ceremony to find a number from 1 to 10 that represents your readiness to proceed to the 2-Week Healing. First, read the example of how one student decided on a number that felt appropriate for her (in the Readiness Check section of this chapter, see comments by participants). Next, it is time to go within and get an assessment number of how ready you actually are.

Close your eyes and pick a number from 1 to 10 that you feel reflects your readiness. Ten means that you are totally ready to move forward (long pause). If you are a 9, work with yourself patiently and with determination (by dialoguing and reviewing) until you are a 10!

If you are in a group, give support to anyone who is in need. It is necessary for everyone in the group to be 100 percent ready before the group can move forward. (Of course, if someone feels absolutely unable to do it even after all kinds of support, she can try again at some later date.)

8. Declarations

Read aloud these statements, written by Dennie LaTourelle and Patricia Bisch:

• *I now let go of fear from all the cells of my body that have been causing me to gain weight, and I replace the fear with total trust in my body to know how to bring me back to my perfect propor-tion. I fill my cells with love. I now let go of guilt and shame from every cell of my body down to the deepest core of what has con-tributed to my food problem. I replace the guilt and shame with self-love, honor and respect for myself, and a knowing that I am enough. (Take a deep breath in and release it.)*

- *I now let go of all anger in the cells of my body that are connected to my food and weight problems. I bring in forgiveness to those I may have hurt unintentionally and to those who may have hurt me unintentionally. I now release all anger for those people who have been involved in my food and weight history, knowing that when we did not feel loved or appreciated we began reacting from a wounded place. (Take a deep breath in and release it.)*

- *I now call back all parts of myself that I have given away or hidden so that I would be loved or not hurt in some way. I call back all of my strength, courage, self-esteem and ability to draw boundaries for myself and say "No" when it is appropriate. I now fully reclaim all of my energy and power. I deeply love myself and stand committed to hold the FFF principles as I return to my perfect proportion. (Take a deep breath in and release it.)*

9. Stating Your Intention

For Individuals: Read aloud the last two paragraphs of your completed individual meditation to affirm your intention to yourself.

For Groups: Stand up in front of the circle and, one by one, read aloud the last two paragraphs of your completed individual meditation to affirm your intention as the group witnesses you. The following is an example:

I know that food of any kind is merely matter or effect and has <u>no power over me</u>. Since Mind is the <u>only Cause</u>, I know that it is <u>only my mental thoughts</u> that can cause bodily effects. I am <u>totally confident</u> that it is not the amount of food, how much food, the times I eat food or the kinds of foods that make me fat. Food <u>cannot cause</u> me to do anything. Food is neutral, nonintentional, mindless energy that has no power over me.

Therefore, I <u>will</u> eat whatever I want, eat as much as I want and not gain weight. I will weigh myself in 2 weeks from when I started, and I will not have gained any weight. I will <u>never gain weight again</u>, no *matter how many days I eat consistently. I am <u>absolutely sure that food does not affect my weight</u>.*

> *I know this is so,*
> *So it is,*
> *Expect a Miracle!!!*
> *Love,*
> _____*(sign your name)*

10. Ending Visualization

Play the tape called Ending Visualization with the *Chariots of Fire* music in the background.

11. Closing

Announcement: In this chapter you are given two additional support meetings that follow this practice session. They will be the guidelines for your next two weekly meetings. Bring food to the next weekly meeting for the Practice Eating and Using the Helpful Hint Tools exercise you will be repeating (see the Chapter 8 practice session). Also bring the Eating at the Ceremony tape and the Ending Visualization tape. Remember to bring a tape recorder and this book to all of the meetings.

For Individuals: You can make an OM sound as you visualize your intentions going out to the universe (optional).

For Groups: Holding hands, just look deeply into each other's eyes, seeing each person empowered and successful. You can make an OM sound as you visualize your intentions going out to the universe (optional). Collect your belongings and leave in silence.

PRACTICE SESSION 9
(additional support meeting #1)

This session is to be held *one week into your 2-Week Healing* and before you weigh in.

Visual Aid: Place all the signs with key words from the previous sessions in front of you as visual reminders of the keys and principles you have learned. For groups, place the words in the center of the circle.

1. Opening Attunement (see sample on p. 13 or p. 14)

If you so desire, light a candle to mark the opening of the session. I recommend that you play the subliminal *Freedom From Food* CD quietly in the background during the attunement.

2. Check-In (2–3 Minutes)

For Individuals: This is an important time to fortify yourself with *only* strong positive thoughts and review the Mastery Keys. Write down in your journal what has been working for you to hold your stand and what you are learning. Remember you are in the consciousness of someone in the Olympics. Looking down at uncomfortable feelings (stomach area) while you are holding a stand will definitely affect your balance. Just tap your Karate Chop Spot if anything makes you nervous.

For Groups: This is an important time to share *only* what is working for you to fortify and hold your stand. Remember your focus must stay up during these 2 weeks. NO doubts or fears at this time. Just tap your Karate Chop Spot if anything makes you nervous. Remember you are in the consciousness of someone in the Olympics. Looking down at uncomfortable feelings (stomach area) will definitely affect your balance. (Be sure to pass the talking piece and use a timer.)

3. Practice Eating

• Do the Practice Eating and Using the Helpful Hint Tools exercise (see the Chapter 8 practice session).

- Play the tape called Eating at the Ceremony while you eat.

- Read testimonials on the 2-Week Healing as a review (see Chapter 9).

- Play Ending Visualization tape as a review.

4. Review the Following Material

a. Read aloud the following story about my own shift (see also Epiphany, Chapter 6)—*When I got on the scale after holding a stand for 2 weeks, I had an "Aha" experience that changed my life forever. To me, looking down at the scale and seeing that I had not gained any weight, after all the junk food I had ingested, was nothing less than a miracle. It was definitely a peak experience in my life! I understood intellectually the steps I had taken to create this, but it still felt like a miracle. This was a life-altering experience. I had read about yogis changing their temperature and doing all kinds of things with their mental focus. However, this was me, Patricia Bisch, changing my body with my focus. I felt empowered and passionately excited.*

By holding onto the new mental focus, I had consciously changed the way food affected my body. I had transmuted incredible amounts of food that I had eaten, food that would have made me gain weight in a day. From a limited linear world of thinking, I had made a quantum shift to a new world with unlimited possibilities concerning food and weight. In this world, I was aligned with universal principles, and I trusted my body's ability to heal. I understood with deep conviction that we live in a world of cocreation between mind and matter, where my thoughts seemed to speed up my metabolism. I understood that my body really is just energy that appears solid. I now knew without a shadow of a doubt that my thoughts could influence my body.

b. Trust and faith about when the shift happens (see Building Trust and Faith, Chapter 8)—People often ask the following question: "When I am holding my stand and my new way of thinking, when does the shift occur that food no longer makes me gain weight?" The answer is "You will not know."

c. Review the section called Thinland (see Chapter 9).

d. Read the quote by Gregg Braden, scientist (see Chapter 4, Using Thoughts to Create Your Reality section).

5. Review the Mastery Keys and Principles (optional)

For Individuals: Write a few sentences in your journal about each one of the following.

For Groups: Share a thought with the group that you remember about each of the following topics:

- Diets Don't Work
- First Mastery Key—The Body Heals Itself
- Second Mastery Key—Mind Creates Matter
- Third Mastery Key—Emotions Affect Your Body
- Fourth Mastery Key—Food Is Energy
- Saboteurs
- Taking a Stand

Reminder for groups: Choose a new leader for the next meeting. Bring food, the Practice Eating at the Ceremony tape and a tape recorder.

6. Appreciation

For Individuals: Write a few sentences in your journal about what most moved or inspired you in this chapter.

For Groups: Go around the circle. Speak about what most moved and inspired you in the meeting today.

7. Closing Attunement (see sample on p. 13 or p. 14)

PRACTICE SESSION 9
(additional support meeting #2)

This session is to be held in the week *immediately after* you weigh in.

Visual Aid: Place all the key words from the previous sessions in front of you as visual reminders of the keys and principles you have learned. For groups, place the key words from previous sessions in the center of the circle.

1. Opening Attunement (see sample on p. 13 or p. 14)

If you so desire, light a candle to mark the opening of the session. I recommend that you play the subliminal *Freedom From Food* CD quietly in the background during the attunement.

2. Check-In (2–3 Minutes)

This is the time to review what has worked for you to hold your stand. First, take a deep breath. Congratulate yourself for completing the 2-Week Healing. It is not uncommon for people to feel somewhat uneasy about holding a new consciousness because it's as if you have moved to a new country. This is a new beginning, and it takes a little time to get used to it.

Take a moment and think about what you have learned from this experience. Most people are amazed that the scale did not move up 5–10 lbs, considering what they have eaten. They are astounded that by aligning their thoughts solidly with the FFF principles, they have changed how their body handles food. People report eating things such as ice cream, hamburgers, french fries, bread and cheese (the taboo binge foods) and not gaining weight. What used to make them gain weight is now going through their system without adding pounds. Many participants say that it feels like a miracle.

Note: If (*and only if*) you have had any problems, see Trouble Shooting After Weighing In, in this practice session, Number 5.

For Individuals: This is an important time to fortify yourself with strong, positive thoughts and to review the Four Mastery Keys. Write down in your journal the amazing discoveries and empowerments you have had during the 2-Week Healing.

For Groups: This is an important time to fortify yourself with strong, positive thoughts and to review the Mastery Keys. Write down in your journal the amazing discoveries and empowerments you have had during the 2-Week Healing. It is not essential for everyone to speak about the outcome of their healing, as this may vary with each person. People with eating problems have been plagued by comparisons and judgments their whole lives. However, it may be positive for one or two people to share success stories. This can create hope, conviction in the process and thoughts of unlimited possibilities for others.

Each group can create its own guidelines concerning this sharing. There are no hard and fast rules. You are like a toddler whose legs are not sturdy; therefore, do not share doubts or fears at this time. It is okay to give reinforcement if someone asks for it, which is different from talking about uncomfortable feelings. For example, a person might ask someone in the group to speak about what makes her feel confident that food will not affect her weight. This is to be distinguished from someone saying, "I don't believe food will not make me gain weight." Just tap your Karate Chop Spot if anything makes you nervous during the sharing. (Be sure to pass the talking piece and use a timer.)

3. Practice Eating

• Practice eating and using the Helpful Hint Tools (see the Chapter 8 practice session).

• Next, play the tape called Eating at the Ceremony while you eat.

4. Review the Mastery Keys and Principles

For Individuals: Write a few sentences about each one in your journals.

For Groups: Write a few sentences about each one in your journals. Speak about what you wrote with the group.

- Diets Don't Work
- First Mastery Key—The Body Heals Itself
- Second Mastery Key—Mind Creates Matter
- Third Mastery Key—Emotions Affect Your Body
- Fourth Mastery Key—Food Is Energy
- Saboteurs
- Taking a Stand

5. Trouble Shooting After Weighing In (Read *only* if you gained weight after the 2-Week Healing.)

If you have gained a couple pounds in the process, don't get down on yourself or panic. It is extremely important to acknowledge what has worked and not start a negative spiral of thinking. Most people can see that although their body/mind may not have completely stopped them from putting on a few pounds, it was successful in decreasing the total amount of weight gain. For example, maybe you gained 2–3 pounds but warded off 7 pounds by holding your focus. It is essential that you give yourself credit where you have been effective.

The next step is to investigate where there is a small leak in your stand or consciousness, where Saboteurs might be gaining ground. Some of the following questions may be helpful:

- Did you entertain negative destructive doubts too long? Did you participate in any conversations that made you uncomfortable concerning weight? Did you visit anyone from the past who has put you down consistently or affected your self-confidence? Did your Saboteurs get to you in some way?

- Did any situations arise that caused a backlash of psychological pain, which may have triggered your need to hold onto weight for protection? Did anything activate old wounds or trauma that you need to talk about with a professional?

- Did you need more protection from your Inner Adult? Did you need help in drawing boundaries or saying "No"?

• Did you hold onto a glance in the mirror, test yourself with clothes to see if they fit or become disturbed by something you read or heard on television?

When you see where there was a leak, make a plan on how you will correct it. Plan what actions you will take to firm up your stand. What will you do differently? The important thing is that you take action right away and do not go into denial.

When you feel you have identified and corrected the problem, go back and do the healing stand again for 3–7 days (or whatever number of days feels like enough time for you to prove to yourself that you will no longer gain weight from food). Repeat exactly what you did in the previous 2-Week Healing. Then get on the scale and see that your weight has remained the same. You will repeat this process until you succeed and your new belief system is holding solidly.

6. Homework

This week, your homework assignment is to do the following:

• Continue eating and holding your new consciousness. Do not weigh yourself now or ever again, unless there is an urgent need for it or if the doctor insists it is necessary for your health in some way. (In 30 years, except when I was pregnant, I have never had a doctor weigh me. When asked, I just say "No," if it is not essential.) Continue reading your meditation and listening to the *Freedom From Food* CD until you feel you do not need it anymore.

Reminder for groups: Choose a new leader for the next meeting. Bring food to the next session to practice eating again.

7. Appreciation

For Individuals: Write a few sentences in your journal about what most moved or inspired you in this chapter.

For Groups: Go around the circle. Speak about what most moved and inspired you in the meeting today.

8. Closing Attunement (see sample on p. 13 or p. 14)

PART V

FOLLOW-UP SUPPORT

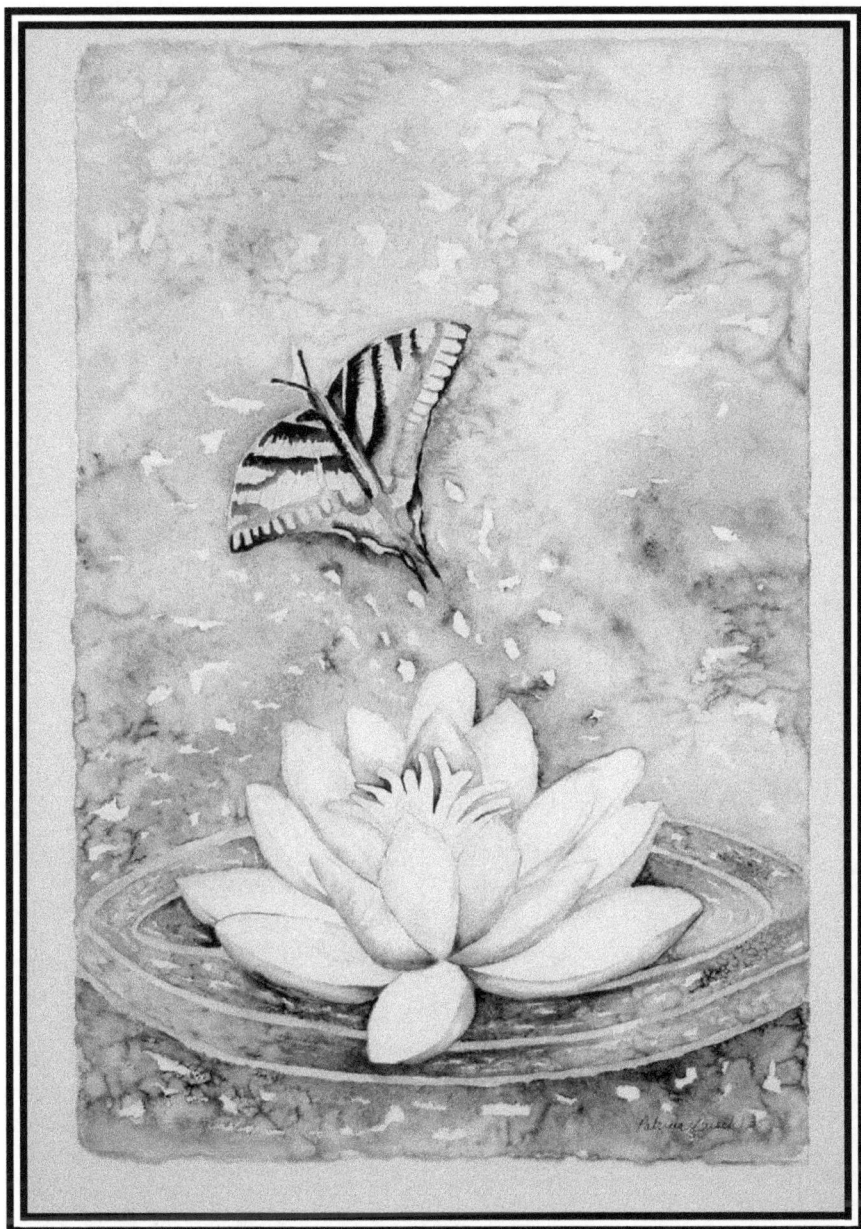

Transformation by Patricia Bisch

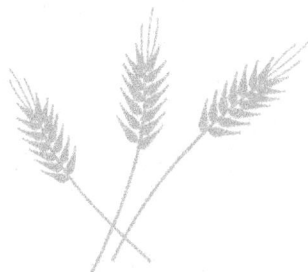

TEN

THE PRACTICE

You can't do it without practice... Until it is fully integrated, you must practice every day...yes, every day. They say it takes a potter years of throwing clay before she can center a pot... It takes a yogi years of discipline and day-to-day practice before she can really do yoga... It takes a martial artist years of constant practice and doing forms before she is a black belt... It takes a dancer years of dancing before she becomes the dance...

—Dennie LaTourelle

The Wise Woman Speaks

Congratulations! It is time to leave the cabin in the forest for your final meeting with the Wise Woman, who is sitting in her favorite chair by the stream. Your seat, graced with a victory garland, is waiting across from her. Looking like a resting tiger, she exudes quiet strength. You have passed successfully through the test of fire, and she is pleased. She knows the trials and tribulations of a Warrioress and what it takes to overcome the dragons of the mind. One last time, the Wise Woman speaks:

Giving yourself credit for your accomplishments is essential to keep your progress in motion. Therefore, take a deep breath and allow all of your cells to bathe in the nourishment of your success, celebrating your transformation.

Like Dorothy in the *Wizard of Oz*, you have found your way back home. You now understand that the answers you seek have always been alive inside of you. The Tin Man learned to understand that he always had a heart and the Scarecrow, that he always had a brain. You also have investigated these parts and used mental prowess to choose only thoughts that create the body you desire. At the same time, you have reconnected with your beautiful heart and emotions, which assisted in healing the pain carried by your Inner Child. For it was the wounds of the heart many years ago that triggered your food problem and the outer search for answers. Finally, like the Lion in the story, you have found courage by calling on your Warrioress to fight Saboteurs. You have amassed the strength necessary to hold a stand and draw firm boundaries around what you believe.

Your changes occurred in the world of fluctuating waves of energy, in which you applied the Ancient Mysteries to the work of manifestation. You have activated the knowledge of how to unite mind and body alchemically to create the perfect proportion you have always wanted.

This is not the end of your journey, however. You are just beginning to enjoy the flow of consciousness you will hold for the rest of your life. It is my wish that you take up permanent residence in Thinland. Both the wisdom to not gain weight from food and the ability to begin losing weight are now awakened in you. It will take continuous, mindful focus until the new ways of thinking are permanently part of the very fabric of your being.

There are no short cuts. Therefore, I respectfully invite you into the final phase of this journey—*the Practice.*

The Practice

The Practice consists of three parts, all of which will require your patience and trust:

- *Part One: Holding the New Consciousness* is about being vigilant in keeping your new consciousness alive and in the forefront of your thinking until it is fully integrated.

• *Part Two: Changing Your Meditation to Include Losing Weight* is about changing your meditation to include phrases that help you begin the process of losing weight.

• *Part Three: Learning About Advanced Eating (My Story)* where you begin to choose and eat foods that improve the quality of your life—that is, selections not based on calories but on how they make you feel.

Part One: Holding the New Consciousness

Although some participants have been healed right after the 2 weeks, most people need ongoing discipline and support over a period of 6 months or more to achieve full integration of their new consciousness. Like a toddler, you may be able to take a few steps, but you may feel safer with something to hold onto at first. It is okay to take additional time and eat a few more hot fudge sundaes, avocados, some bread and butter or whatever it is until you feel assured that you will not gain weight from any food. Going through more situations and testing out your newfound abilities will solidify the potency of your stand. Complete all the possibilities until your mind surrenders and lets go of all old, masquerading doubts. When you have no more entangled or distorted thoughts, you can proceed with losing weight.

The process of mastering the FFF concepts is like learning to ride a bike. At first, it is hard to find your balance. You must remember all the moves so you don't fall off. This extreme concentration can create a subtle contraction in your body/mind. Then one day, the process is integrated. You maintain a relaxed balance without even thinking about it and no longer need training wheels. Riding the bike becomes automatic—you just do it!

Another example of the kind of mastery needed can be observed in students who are studying martial arts. Their training includes poses or forms practiced repeatedly to instill a higher state of body/mind awareness. If you observe a black-belt martial artist, you will notice that her moves seem effortless. Although she has endured many hours of concentrated practice to become proficient, she has no intention of fighting. However, in an instant, if a threatening situation arises and some Saboteurs show up, she is prepared to defend herself.

In the following practice sessions, you will find the support to fully embody the FFF principles at a black-belt level. There will come a time when you no longer need the assistance of your meditation, Helpful Hint Tools and so on. You will have moved permanently to Thinland and be living like those who know without a shadow of a doubt that food is not connected to weight.

Note: Your program may need to be personalized by modification and supplementation with professional help, such as EFT, EMDR, hypnosis, medical treatment and so on. The process varies with each individual, and it is important to honor your unique path.

Part Two: Changing Your Meditation to Include Losing Weight

When you have successfully completed your 2-Week Healing and feel confident that food does not affect your weight, it is time to change your meditation to carry the intention to *lose weight*. The details of how to do this are in the practice session that follows.

This part of the healing is *not done in any specific timeframe*, such as a 2-Week Healing. In my experience, releasing weight happens primarily by holding onto the principles. Then at a point when you *don't even know it*, you will be *losing weight*. As I have mentioned before, no one knows the exact moment this will take place. Just as you cannot open up the cocoon of the caterpillar before it becomes the butterfly, you cannot check on whether or not you are losing weight. This will disturb and maybe destroy the birth you are giving. Don't forget that your body is always attempting to go to its highest state of health (which includes attaining your ideal weight). If you just let it do its job, your body will astound you!

Participant's Comment After 2-Week Healing

About a month after the 2-Week Healing, which I completed and did not gain weight, I went on a 2-month trip to Europe with a friend of mine—believe me, we ate our way around Europe. We had a big breakfast every day, a big lunch, a huge dinner with wine, and no day went by without afternoon pastries. This trip has since been called "my celebratory binge around Europe." Upon my return to America, I weighed myself. My friend had gained 12 pounds on the trip, and I had LOST 17 pounds! I have never weighed myself since.

Part Three: Learning About Advanced Eating

When I first healed myself, I was still getting over my years of food addiction and deprivation. Although I was no longer gaining weight and I had lost weight, I was still at times covering up pain and anxiety by overeating. I was conscious of how food affected my weight but very out of touch with its influence on my energy level, clarity or mood.

Awhile after my 2-Week Healing, I began to feel calmer when thinking about food, and the feeling of deprivation was fading away. I was no longer a prisoner of my compulsion, because I was now able to eat anything and not gain weight. Therefore, a space opened up for me to actually feel whether my body was happy with my choices. This was the beginning of the stage I call *Advanced Eating*. The numbness caused by overeating had worn off, and I could not stuff myself without being aware of the horrible price I was paying.

No longer oblivious, I was able to start referencing specifically what happened to my body as I ate certain foods. For example, did I become more tired or less clear? I began to see how having ice cream before bedtime affected my energy level, making me sluggish and foggy the next day. For the first time in my life, I felt that I could freely *choose* to eat something based on how it would affect me. Now I could substitute fruit or health bars for cookies and candy.

If you eat chocolate cake all the time, you eventually will want something different—whether it is a sandwich, salad or so forth. I have observed that people really do want to feel better. An innate yearning naturally emerges and leads them to make choices that enhance their well-being. If an apple makes you feel better than a candy bar, over time you will choose the apple. When this starts to happen it is a sign that you are entering the stage of Advanced Eating. At this time it is good to affirm all new behaviors to strengthen them.

Here are some examples of what you might say: "With each choice I make, I create more energy in my body and greater clarity in my mind." "Because I love myself, I am choosing to eat what enhances my well-being." "With each Advanced Eating choice I make, my body is healthier and functions more harmoniously."

Most likely, you will still on occasion eat things that do not make you feel great the next day. Once in a while, you may emotionally eat if you feel bored, unloved, angry or frustrated. You might also eat more during a special occasion. However, despite these times, you will continue a natural course toward better and better health without putting on extra pounds.

Trouble Shooting

(Read *only* if you are having difficulties with the program.)

If you are having difficulty holding this new FFF consciousness and not gaining weight, it is important to read the following information. You may be letting sabotaging thoughts come in, many of which you are not aware. Definitely reread Chapter 7 and Chapter 8. If you are putting on extra pounds and think it is not just your sabotaging thoughts or doubting voices (be careful, they are tricky), *stop right away* and begin to assess what is going on. You may require medical help or some other form of professional guidance. You may not be able to figure it out alone and that is perfectly okay. Remember this saying: "Insanity is doing the same thing over and over again and expecting different results" (attributed to Albert Einstein).

Although you are not supposed to check to see if you are gaining weight during and after the 2-Week Healing (the watched pot never boils), there may come a point where you have sufficient evidence to question whether the process needs to be adjusted. Has more than a week or two gone by and your clothes really don't fit? Do you feel you *definitely* have gained weight and it is not just a temporary shapeshift? Begin by asking the following questions that may show you a way to tighten up your stand:

• Have you used all of your Helpful Hint Tools and your body is still not adjusting?

• Could the problem be medical? Have you stopped or started some new medication? How is your thyroid or hormones? I recommend that you check with a medical doctor.

• Are you eating foods to which you could be allergic? Do you have wheat or milk intolerance? Have you checked for Candida or other conditions?

• Is it your thinking? Have you gone back to believing that food, fasting, cleansing, exercise or something else will make you lose weight? Have you noticed that you have *temporarily* fallen into some old landmines of negative ideas and are not feeling good about your body?

• Have you been getting the support you need?

• Is there a psychological issue? Has something happened recently that has triggered wounds from the past and your Inner Child is using your body to protect you by keeping weight on? Do you need to do some more trauma work with a professional?

• Have you prematurely stopped doing things that helped you not gain weight during the 2-Week Healing, such as listening to the CDs or reading your FFF meditation?

First try to remedy the problem and do the stand again. In my experience, you will most likely succeed. Do not go on eating whatever you want if your consciousness is not clear or your body is having a negative reaction. You should absolutely not be gaining weight at this point. If you cannot resolve the difficulty, it may be necessary to add or modify this program with some other way of controlling your weight. In extreme cases it may be necessary to stop the program completely. It is important not to blame yourself or someone else. Be gentle with yourself as you keep moving forward to discover your next step.

Reinforcing the Stand

My message for the next months is to *practice, practice and practice* while holding your new consciousness. Then one day, when you are not even thinking about it, it will just be a part of you. Like the very air you breathe, food will come in and go out of your system unobstructed by your mind.

As you begin to realize that food will not affect your body negatively, you can begin to relax. You will become as confident that your body will eliminate excess calories as you are that your heart will beat. Simultaneously, your Inner Child will deepen her connection to her Inner Adult. Food will no longer need to be the glue that holds your fragmented parts together. Eating will be replaced by an uninterrupted flow of love running through your veins, allowing you to feel safer in this world.

As you practice FFF over the next months, be mindful of the following helpful coaching tips:

Patience. Impatience is the number-one killer of this program. It is the sabotaging part within that convinces us we cannot go with our natural flow and timing to incorporate the ideas we have learned. It says we have to go on a diet and lose weight now. Out of desperation, we superimpose a limited timeframe on ourselves rather than deeply listen to the natural pace of our body while it makes its adjustments.

This need to rush creates self-induced amnesia. We forget all of the ineffective, fast-moving diets we have tried. Expecting impossible deadlines, we brutally and intolerantly tell ourselves that we must fit into a new bathing suit or special dress by some unrealistic date. We decide to do a quick diet or cleanse to lose weight faster, thinking we will get right back on the FFF program when it is over. If this kind of thinking sounds like you, here's a warning. The saboteurs will be looming outside your door, ready to strip you of all you have attained —until they see that you leave no opening to be preyed upon. It is only then that they will lose interest.

Take a moment and reflect on your state of mind. Ask yourself the following questions:

- Are you experiencing impatience that causes you to forget the trauma, terror and events you have endured to get to this point?

- Does your attitude honor you for the months you have put into this program?

- Are you losing patience with yourself for the time it takes to heal the emotional issues connected to your weight, so you will no longer have to protect yourself with food?

If your answer is "Yes" to any of these questions, remember this: If you retreat from your goal, it can be extremely difficult to create a firm stand once again. It is therefore important to *guard against interrupting the process.*

When you feel impatient, take a moment and affirm, "I trust my body's perfect timing," or "Whether I can see it or not, I know that I am already in process of returning to my perfect proportion" or "I have all the patience I need to allow my body to heal itself."

It is good to be gentle and loving with yourself, willing to allow whatever time it takes to banish your extra pounds. Although you may feel this is hard to do and will take forever, healing can actually occur very quickly. There is a mystery in all of this. Reread Gregg Braden's quote (in the Chapter 4 section called Using Thoughts to Create Your Reality), in which he describes a healing that took place in 2 minutes and 40 seconds. Your thoughts, beliefs and emotions are powerful!!! You can do this.

Maintaining Trust. To maintain trust at this time, it is essential for you to reexamine many of the concepts from the previous chapters and give yourself ongoing support. An in-depth review is outlined in the practice session that follows. For example,

- (Review Homeostasis in Chapter 3)—It is important to maintain trust beyond any *temporary* appearances in the body, since there is a natural ebb and flow that happens in our physical form. Water levels, temperature levels and sugar levels are just a few things that are constantly changing. Our bodies do not exist in a straight line. Perfect proportion is maintained through the fluctuations and variations that occur all the time. Our bodies are naturally self-correcting organisms. There is balance and homeostasis inherent in the system.

- (Review Learning to Trust in Chapter 3)—If your body has the appearance of gaining weight during fluctuations from salt intake, hormones, menstrual cycle or sick thinking, for example, you will need to go into trust. You do not have to know how or when your body will self-correct and balance out. You just need to have faith that it will do so. Remember, in a day or two after you are full from a meal, the fullness is always gone. *Your body takes care of it,* and you don't have to know how. Doubting consciousness blocks up the energy flow. Just take your attention off what is happening and trust that in one or two days, the problem is usually gone.

- (Review Food and Air in Chapter 6)—A brownie has no more power over you than a carrot stick. In the FFF paradigm, they are both mindless energy that would go right through you if you did not interfere in the process with your beliefs.

Just Say 'No'

After my 2-Week Healing, my mental practice was one of never going back to the inner hell, the roller coaster of dieting and gaining weight that I had lived with for so many years. I vowed that I would never open the door to that line of thinking again and would do whatever it took to uphold my new beliefs about food. If put to the test, I would say "No" to any alluring kind of deprivation (fad diets, cleanses, exercise programs to lose weight, etc.). Instead, I would intentionally continue eating whatever I wanted.

Sometimes, when I first started my practice, I would look down and think that I saw weight. I might see a roll of fat that I didn't remember being there, or at times, I just felt that I looked larger. With panic building, my mind would say, "You need to diet now!!! You need to lose this weight." I would witness my mind thinking panic thoughts and hear fear from this part of me. What worked was to shift my mind away from listening to these mental Saboteurs. I knew they were trying to call me back to my old way of dieting and deprivation.

I replaced these negative thoughts with thoughts that I repeated over and over again about trusting my body's intelligence. I had faith that my body inherently knew how to eliminate anything that was toxic or unnecessary for me. I had just proven that to myself in the 2-Week Healing. Nevertheless, I needed to keep up my practice of holding my new FFF consciousness. I understood that I hadn't yet solidly integrated the principles to the place where I had no doubt. I still had some sick thinking, not knowing if I was thin enough.

However, my commitment paid off, and there did come a time when my practice was totally integrated and my Inner Saboteurs gave up. I had won the battle, as Eckhart Tolle has said, and I was able to walk the tightrope of consciousness with total focus. As a result, the little voices had nothing to hold onto. I had developed relentless, unshakable faith in my body's ability to keep itself in perfect proportion.

I am now a black-belt in regard to food. I eat and live as a thin person with the complete knowing that no matter how much I eat, I never gain weight. Although I seem totally carefree in this area, I have an impenetrable boundary around me to any sabotaging thoughts that try to come in. I have no intention of ever letting something take me back to my old way of thinking and the desperate life I was living.

For a while, however, the past seemed to be just a thought away. People would come with all kinds of questions, advice, doubts, new facts, programs and fears. I never let them in. Now these temptations can't even get close to me. I have been totally free from food for over 30 years with no deprivation. I have no need to question, prove or think that I need some other point of view. This has given me my entrance to Thinland with the total freedom to eat whatever I want. Now food is just a wonderful part of my life that I enjoy!

Parting Reflections From the Author

In the end, on an emotional level, it is all about love and valuing oneself. All of the wounds that you have endured in this life have an effect on your heart and body. For most of us, these were so painful and frightening that we felt there was no choice but to close down for protection. Food was the vehicle we used to survive. It numbs pain and creates some semblance of short-term safety. However, then you are left with loneliness, separation and anxiety created by closing and walling off your heart.

Years later, I still get brief reminders of how I used to live before I moved to Thinland. Certain experiences bring up the wounds, pains, hurt and feelings of being unloved that I once endured. These reappearances keep me grateful and remembering that I have been given a second chance to have my life. They are flashbacks that help reinforce the importance of never taking my healing for granted. It just takes a moment for me to shift if I reflect on the futility of staying on a diet, how much deprivation it caused and how quickly the weight came rushing back.

The old patterns show up especially when I feel upset over something. It is usually still about a man in my life (my father wound). I sometimes reach for food to soothe myself. It's not about a whole bag of food, it doesn't go on for days and I don't ever gain weight. I might eat a half pint of ice cream or some candy, but food never takes over my life. I can now laugh compassionately and sweetly instead of loathing and hating myself.

Keeping on track is much easier because I don't gain weight anymore. I am aware that food represents giving myself something emotionally when I am not getting the love I need, when worried about losing the love I have or when anxious about never having the love I want. A friend will call me, and I tell her I am eating a pint of ice cream and I am upset at some situation. Admitting what I am doing is no longer shameful to me because I am not perpetually at the mercy of my compulsion. We laugh, and I tell her about my anxiety. These days, with the work I've done on myself, that's usually all it takes.

I don't do long binges anymore or indulge in liquor store stops. Mostly, I eat foods that keep my energy up and my mind clear—the Advanced Eating way. I do every once in a while give myself an ice cream bar, multiple desserts at a buffet, as much Halloween candy as I want or something like that. It's OK, and I thoroughly enjoy my splurge. The one law I keep solidly is never to stop myself from eating in any way that makes me feel the slightest bit deprived. If I am tempted to deprive myself, I eat whatever I am afraid of. This keeps me free and out of the futile world of diets.

The war, the wounds, the deep separation and feeling unloved are over. My healing began with my story about my father, when he withdrew his love and I lost my self-worth and value. I thought I would never be happy again. It is no surprise that this conclusion to my book mentions how I have healed my father wound and found my value. It's funny, but without purposely doing it, I am writing this on his birthday. It has been a long journey, and I am crying a little as I write. I wish he could have been alive for this time when I found myself. I wish he could have healed himself enough to celebrate me. Even though he is not alive, I talked to him today. In some place deep inside, I felt like he was watching and smiling.

I now understand that the love from a man never really had anything to do with looks. As hard as I tried to be pretty, that still didn't get me what I wanted. It was only when I valued myself in the highest way that I could receive love. It came as a reflection of myself.

I love myself now. There is a warm, compassionate feeling in my heart. I can see my incredible strengths and my weaknesses. There have been passages through dark nights of the soul, revisiting some horrible places. Yet, what remains is my deep gratitude and amazement for the miracle that has happened.

I hope that this program will be the final stop in your healing process, or that it has given you some essential tools to venture forth on another path that feels right for you. You are forming a new relationship with food and yourself. This is an ongoing process of upgrading your food and your thinking for the rest of your life. It takes whatever time it takes. Keep on peeling off the layers of the problem until the last layer is gone and you are at the weight you want to be. Never give up. In the end, food is actually a sacred substance. It is not only here for us to enjoy, but more important, it is also the manna or energy Mother Earth has supplied to sustain and nourish us. I now deeply understand that it is only energy, and it really never was my enemy.

Holding a stand gives you an opportunity to see and value yourself for the strength and guts of who you are. You have been love from the very beginning. In truth, that is all you will ever be. Just as the dancer becomes the dance, I wish for you to become one with your body's natural healing system. May this program be a road back home to yourself, leading to its perfect reflection in your body temple.

And now, take a moment to put your hand gently on your heart, open, breathe and congratulate yourself for all that you have done to get this far. You have everything you need to reclaim your beautiful body and the life you want now! I have full trust in the powerful, radiant Warrioress who lives inside of you. It is time to let yourself shine in your full magnificence and be all that you were always meant to be.

Thank you for journeying with me into the magic and wonder of bringing the formless into form.

Patricia Bisch

(The Wise Woman who exists within all of us)

PRACTICE SESSION 10
WEEKLY SUPPORT GROUPS

This practice session is the model for all future meetings. It differs in several ways from previous ones. For example, in Step 8 of the session, you will *choose* a different weekly topic to reexamine rather than being assigned one. You are not complete with the course even though you have gone through the 2-week healing. To create a solid, lasting stand, it is necessary to attend two months of support meetings. In fact, I highly recommend 6 months.

Visual Aid: On a piece of paper, write the following key words and place them as a visual reminder in front of you. For groups, place this paper in the center of the circle. For this chapter, the sign will say:

~ Put in Whatever You Choose as the Weekly Topic ~

1. Opening Attunement (see sample on p. 13 or p. 14)

If you so desire, light a candle to mark the opening of the session. I recommend that you play the subliminal *Freedom From Food* CD quietly in the background during the attunement.

2. Check-In (2–3 Minutes)

For Individuals: Write a page or more in your journal as a check-in with yourself. What is working for you to maintain your new FFF consciousness?

For Groups: Allow a 2–3-minute check-in per person. This should mainly focus on the positive and what is working for you to maintain your new FFF consciousness. Rather than voicing your doubts and fears, ask for reinforcement when you need it. Remember to tap your Karate Chop Spot if someone is sharing something and you begin to feel uncomfortable. You can just tap it without thinking about anything in particular, which will keep out unwanted thoughts. People have reported feeling better simply by taking this action. Also, share any new insights you have had during the week. (Remember to pass the talking piece and use a timer.)

3. 5-Minute Sharing

For Individuals: Take this time to read something that reinforces your new consciousness. You can use information from one of the chapters or outside material that is compatible. Write down any new insights in your journal.

For Groups: This is a special time for one person (per session) to speak about what has been working in this program. You can also use this time to ask for reinforcement in any area. For example, if you need help to remember why cookies will not cause weight gain, it's OK to ask others what they are doing that is beneficial. This process will strengthen everyone.

4. Appreciations

For Individuals: This is a good time to write down three appreciations of yourself—something about your essence. See the examples that follow.

For Groups: Three people from the group can give brief appreciations for the person who has just spoken. An appreciation should be something about the person's essence—what you notice about that person. An appreciation should not give advice or include an explanation about how the person's story relates to your story. Here are some examples of the kinds of appreciations you might offer:

I love your courage and the way you speak up for yourself.
I appreciate how you protect your Inner Child.
I think you are radiant, and I love the way you light up when you smile.

5. Break

6. Change Your Meditation

Change One: If you have successfully completed your 2-Week Healing without gaining weight, it is now time to add some new proofs to your daily meditation. You will now include some examples of what you ate during the 2-Week Healing. For example, you may have eaten lots of ice cream and bread and butter one day and your body didn't put on extra pounds. Here is an example of how to add a new paragraph:

From my 2-Week Healing, I now know that food does not make me gain weight. For during the 2 weeks, I ate lots of ice cream and bread and butter...and I did not gain weight.

Add several more examples, which will empower your stand and make it even stronger. Continue reading the whole meditation every day for as long as you feel you need it. This will fortify and add credibility to yourself that food no longer affects you in the same way. Remember, do not get on the scale!

Change Two: When you feel integrated and confident in your new belief system that food will not make you gain weight, you are ready to begin losing weight! Don't rush the process. It may take a few weeks or months to feel strong in your new consciousness. The timing will be different for each person, and it is important to honor your own pace.

To begin the process of losing weight, you need to change the words in the last paragraph of your meditation. Replace the words "and I will not gain weight" with the words "and I am losing weight now." (Do not get on the scale again!! It is not necessary because you already weighed at the end of the 2-Week Healing.) Continue reading this revised meditation 10 minutes a day for as long as you need it. Also continue using whatever tools contributed to your success during the 2-week stand. Here is an example of how to change the last paragraph in your meditation:

Therefore, I will eat whatever I want, eat as much as I want and I will lose weight. I am returning to my perfect proportion. I know that I will never gain weight again, no matter how many days I eat consistently. I am absolutely sure that food does not affect my weight and that I am losing weight now.

I know this is so,

So it is,

Expect a Miracle!!!

Love,

_____ *(sign your name)*

This part of the healing is *not done in any timeframe*, such as a 2-Week Healing. In my experience, losing weight happens just by holding onto the principles, and then at a point when you *don't even know it*, you will be *losing weight*. Be patient, *don't check, let go; trust* your body to naturally take you back to your perfect proportion.

If you just let it do its job, your body will amaze you!!! Therefore, just keep holding these thoughts impeccably in your mind and the subatomic particles will be affected in your body. Keep up your weekly practice and trust!! (Review Testimonials, p. 1.)

7. Practice Eating Exercise

Throughout the weeks to come, it will be good reinforcement to continue practicing eating while using the Helpful Hints Tools. (For details, review Practice Eating and Using the Helpful Hints Tools in the Chapter 8 practice session).

8. Recommended Topics for Your Ongoing Weekly Practice

Each week, scan the following topics and choose the one that seems most pertinent to address. While groups can share and discuss the topic in the circle, individuals can write down thoughts in their journals. Reviewing any of the material you have studied, redoing practice sessions and introducing supportive material from outside sources all provide beneficial weekly subjects. The suggested discussion topics that follow are not to be used in any particular order. Most of them will be a review.

a. Maintain Trust. It is important to maintain trust beyond temporary appearances in your body, since there is a *natural ebb and flow that happens* in physical form. Perfect proportion is maintained through the fluctuations and variations that occur all the time. Our bodies are naturally self-correcting organisms (see sections on Homeostasis and Trust in Chapter 3).

b. Shapeshifting Is Possible. If you have temporarily fallen into old land mines of negative thinking and are not feeling good about your body, remember that shapeshifting is possible. Healing can take place in an instant when intention and conviction are present. Review the reports from participants on how they successfully did it (see Shapeshifting section in Chapter 4).

c. Avoid the Mirror. As overeaters, we have been sick thinkers about our weight. Much of what we think we see is an illusion. We often think we are fat when we are not. We have distorted images of ourselves. Much like anorexic people, those with weight problems lose perspective of how their body really looks. That is why it is so important not to use the mirror as you would a scale.

Many participants shared the experience of thinking that they were fat as children. However, now when they look back at pictures of themselves at a young age, they realize they were really not over-weight at all or certainly not to the degree they remembered. Their visual perception was tainted by other people's projected thoughts, comparisons and opinions that became internalized as fact.

If you happen to look at yourself in the mirror and think you have gained weight, it is important not to take this perception as a solid fact. Remember, people were absolutely sure the world looked flat until Magellan sailed around it. Our perceptions can be mislead-ing. Also, our vision tells us our world is solid matter when the truth is that it is energy slowed down to appear like mass.

For all of these reasons, many participants continued covering their mirrors for months after the 2-Week Healing. In some instances, they left an opening just for their face. This helped them not make conclusions about temporary illusions, which gave their bodies time to rearrange.

d. Release Scale Consciousness—Don't Check. Checking comes in many forms. All of these are lethal to your success and will break your stand. Your saboteurs will create convincing and compelling reasons why you must check to see if you are gaining weight. They will feed you statements such as the following: "You have no choice. You have nothing to wear. You have to see if some of your old clothes fit." (Review this list in Chapter 8, Building Trust and Faith section.)

The scale is like a roller coaster that creates diet consciousness. It fluctuates so much and does not give your body time to rearrange to your new "perfectly proportioned" mental image. Therefore, I recommend that you wear baggy clothes that are loose so you do not micromanage yourself. Give the seeds you plant time to grow without pulling them up to check.

Also, many people use feeling into their body like they would use a scale. They say they know for certain whether they have put on extra pounds by how their body feels. They take this feeling measurement as absolute truth. However, in my experience, they are often wrong. This kind of checking may cause a break in focus that creates doubt.

e. Think of Thinland. (review section on Thinland, Chapter 9).

f. Take a Risk. Do something to get more into life. Put your attention on making your life the exciting and fulfilled one you've always wanted. Are you expressing your unique gifts? Maybe it is time to begin doing the things you have always wanted to try but didn't seem to have the courage to start. Remember the words of Georgia O'Keefe, the great artist: "I'm frightened all the time… scared to death. But I've never let it stop me. Never!" (Access at: www. hanksville.org)

Discuss where in your life you need to stretch and expand to be more of the incredible, unique person you are. You may have to walk through a little fear now. Behind the fear is usually excitement. When you are risking, you are not bored, doing the status quo. Stop waiting (weighting).

Most people who have lost weight on this program say that it happened when they got more into life and stopped thinking about their food problem. Do things that you have always wanted to do, such as taking a computer class, dance lessons, singing, public speaking, acting or art. Remember, when you start flowing in life, it creates movement on the inside. Stuck places that are contracted begin to let go. It's time now to go for it and be the person you've always wanted to be!

g. Go Over the Mastery Keys and Principles. Review the principles from each chapter and write a few sentences about each one. Discuss them in your group if you have one.

h. Practice Patience. Patience is required. You need to be gentle and loving with yourself. Impatience is the number-one killer of this program. Each individual's timing will be unique. You must honor your own path (see Patience, this chapter).

i. Speed up Your Metabolism. Have another magazine day and cut out different pictures that reflect the body you would like to have. Visualization can send the message to your body metabolism to speed up and return to its perfect proportion (see Homework in the Chapter 6 practice session).

j. Share Articles and Books That Support Your New Consciousness. Read inspiring books or articles that support your new FFF consciousness. In your own practice, bring in something every day that enlivens your thoughts and inspires you. If you are looking to substantiate your new consciousness, the right people, situations, books and articles will come your way. This is the law of attraction. If you are in a group, bring in all supportive materials to share.

k. Use a Buddy System.

For Groups: Choose a buddy to call weekly. Check in with them for positive reinforcement only. These calls are not for the purpose of sharing sabotaging fears or doubts. If you tend to be a people pleaser, here is a chance to assert yourself. Do not listen if the information being shared starts throwing you off center. Stop the conversation immediately and gently remind your buddy to phrase things more positively. Share with each other the practices you are doing daily to affirm your stance and keep it going.

l. Tapping Rounds. As a group or individually, you may decide that you need a chance to get rid of some build-up of negative thinking. I recommend that you do this whenever you feel it is necessary. However, don't forget to add the positive phrase at the end of all your statements (review Tap Your Saboteurs Away section in Chapter 7).

m. Mindfulness. (referred to in Buddhist traditions). Mindfulness is an important process in dealing with your thoughts. In regard to this program, it is about being very watchful about which thoughts you entertain and which ones you let pass on through. For some people, it takes only one absolutely negative thought said with conviction (even if it is wrong) to create a change in body weight. That's why so many people say they can just look at food and gain weight. The good news is that replacing it with a positive thought is equally potent to produce weight loss. Remember that your mind is the commander and chief controller of the energy that composes your body form. You *do* have the free will to choose and be vigilant about the thoughts you entertain.

Be mindful and do not bypass even one traumatic incident of looking in the mirror and thinking you have gained weight. You must replace all of these kinds of thoughts right away with more positive ones.

It is your certainty that accompanies a false belief that is a large part of the problem. Often what you see can be a false illusion, which is really bloat or a feeling of fullness that will go away. If you are not telling yourself that what you perceive as weight gain has at least the *possibility* of being a temporary false perception, you are in trouble. There must be some part of yourself that will question what you see. Even when I lost weight and was very thin, I still imagined that I was too heavy. As eaters, we do not always have an accurate view of ourselves. Therefore, investigate the truth behind your thoughts before you accept them.

Reminder for groups: Choose a new leader for the next meeting. Bring food, the Practice Eating at the Ceremony tape and a tape recorder.

9. Appreciation

For Individuals: Write a few sentences in your journal about what most moved or inspired you in this chapter.

For Groups: Go around the circle. Speak about what most moved and inspired you in the meeting today.

10. Closing Attunement (see sample on p. 13 or p. 14)

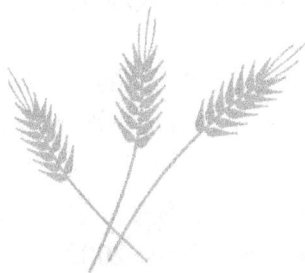

BIBLIOGRAPHY

Arenson, Gloria. *Five Simple Steps to Emotional Healing: The Last Self-Help Book You Will Ever Need.* Simon & Schuster, 2001.

Aurobindo. *The Mother.* Sri Aurobindo Ashram, 1972.

Bandler, Richard, and Grinder, John. *Frogs Into Princes: Neuro Linguistic Programming.* Real People Press, 1979.

Braden, Gregg. *The Isaiah Effect: Decoding the Lost Science of Prayer and Prophecy.* Three Rivers Press, 2000.

Chopra, Deepak. *Perfect Weight: The Complete Mind-Body Program for Achieving and Maintaining Your Ideal Weight.* Harmony Books, 1994.

Cohen, Harvey. *The Incredible Credible Cosmic Consciousness Diet for Weight Loss and World Peace.* Aa Ha! Dynamics Press, 1984.

Cole-Whittaker, Terry. *What You Think of Me Is None of My Business.* Oak Tree Publishing, 1979.

Emoto, Masuro. *Messages From Water: World's First Pictures From Water Crystals.* HADO Kyoikusha Co.

Fox, Emmet. *Power Through Constructive Thinking.* Harper Brothers, 1932.

Hendricks, Gay. *Conscious Breathing: Breathwork for Health, Stress Release and Personal Mastery.* Bantam, 1995.

Levine, Peter, and Frederick, Ann. *Waking the Tiger: Healing Trauma: The Innate Capacity to Transform Overwhelming Experiences.* North Atlantic Books, 1997.

Paul, Margaret, and Chopich, Erika J. *Healing Your Aloneness: Finding Love and Wholeness Through Your Inner Child.* Harper San Francisco, 1990.

Pearce, Joseph Chilton. *The Biology of Transcendence: A Blueprint of the Human Spirit.* Park Street Press, 2002.

Pert, Candace B. *Molecules of Emotion: Why You Feel the Way You Feel.* Scribner, 1997.

Pert, Candace B., with Nancy Marriott. *Everything You Need to Know to Feel Go(o)d.* Hay House, 2006.

Ray, Sondra. *The Only Diet There Is.* Celestial Arts, 1981.

Roth, Geneen. *When Food Is Love: Exploring the Relationship Between Eating and Intimacy.* Plume, 1992.

Simonton, O. Carl. *Getting Well Again.* J. P. Tarcher, 1978.

Tolle, Eckhart. *The Power of Now: A Guide to Spiritual Enlightenment.* New World Library, 2004.

Williamson, Marianne. *A Return to Love: Reflections on the Principles of "A Course in Miracles."* Harper Collins, 1992.

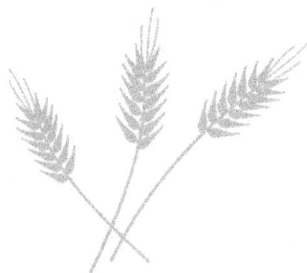

ABOUT THE AUTHOR

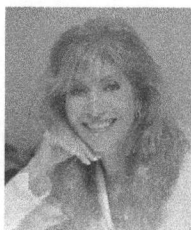

Patricia Bisch, MA, MFT, lived the painful life of an overeater from her teen years to well into early adulthood. Then, over 30 years ago, she discovered the secret to regaining her power over food—not through deprivation, but as a way to enjoy eating and to lose weight anyway. She proceeded to practice and perfect the principles she writes about, and today, she remains completely healed. In addition to reaching master-level proficiency in two energetic healing methods and maintaining a private practice in psychotherapy, Patricia lectures, conducts media appearances and leads classes and workshops on weight loss. She lives, writes and creates her audio CDs in southern California where she is a healthy, vibrant, living advertisement for the benefits of gaining Freedom From Food.

PURCHASE *FREEDOM FROM FOOD* CDS ON THE INTERNET

You can purchase a set of CDs to support your success in the Freedom From Food program. The two CDs are as follows:

Audible CD with Music in 3 Parts:

1. Guided Visualizations, incorporating the FFF principles of how to eat whatever you want and not gain weight
2. Affirmations for Healing
3. Healing Your Inner Child

Subliminal CD with Music in 3 Parts: Uses the same 3 parts as in the audible CD, but the words are programmed into the CD below the level of sound. You hear only the music and your subconscious hears the words. This creates a powerful support to help you hold your new consciousness about food while you relax or go about other activities.

To Order: Simply visit **cdbaby.com**. Go to search and type in Freedom From Food or speak to a real live person by calling this toll-free number: (800) 289-6923. All major credit cards accepted; purchases shipped within hours of your order.

> My "Aha!" moment came when I was listening to the guided visualization on the audible *FFF* CD. I saw in my mind how food breaks down to tiny subatomic particles and then interacts with the body. This helped me to shift from seeing food as fat and calories that cause weight to seeing food for what it really is: tiny units of energy that are nourishing my body. *From that moment, I was free from all my old ideas that food makes me fat!*
>
> —Participant

FREEDOM FROM FOOD LECTURES, EVENTS AND CONTACTS

Visit www.PatriciaBisch.com

www.ingramcontent.com/pod-product-compliance
Lightning Source LLC
Chambersburg PA
CBHW031505270326
41930CB00006B/251